# BBQ

## FISH & VEGETABLES

## Special Edition

Easy and Delicious Recipes:

Salmon, Shrimp, Tuna, Tilapia, Halibut, Octopus, Lobster and many Vegetables Recipes.

Bruno Montana

# TABLE OF CONTENTS

# THE BENEFITS OF BARBEQUE GAS GRILLS

Gas grills work by a spark igniting the gas within the grill. Gas grills typically have a knob or button in which you push, which activates a small hammer. The hammer hit is the top of an ignition crystal. Then the burner mixes the gas with oxygen and spreads it all over the cooking surface.

Barbequing is typically thought of as a summer event, but some diehard fans of barbeque will not think twice about breaking out their barbeque grills right in the middle of Winter. Grillers in the southern states may not face the problem, but if you live past the lower States, then chances are your Winter includes a large amount of snow. Smokers and charcoal grills present a problem as you must set the grill up correctly and then wait for the grill to get ready. This can take hours, so the idea of standing outside waiting on the grill may not sound appealing in 3 feet of snow. Gas grills allow you to quickly cooking barbeque.

Another issue found without types of grills is the cleanup involved. Once you are done grilling with a smoker or charcoal grill, you must clean out the burned remains. In 3 feet of snow, the chances are that you do not have a place readily available for disposal. Fire hazards come with the burnt coals and wood chips. Gas grills will need a wipe down before they can be stored away for the next time.

Unlike some of the other grills types, gas grills can come with many different types of cooking surfaces. These different cooking surfaces include a BBQ surface, a flat grill, and a ribbed grill. Some grills even offer these types of surfaces as none stick, which allow you to cook a whole array of foods that you would not be able to cook on a grill otherwise. You will be able to cook your complete meal, including side dishes if you plan correctly. Some gas grills even contain a Wok-type surface for cooking pasta and rice dishes or a complete rotisserie set that allows you to cook rotisserie chicken.

A feature that comes with different cooking surfaces is the ability to cook other foods, at different temperatures, at the same time. This feature is available if your gas grill has separate burners. This allows you to cook your meals much more quickly. Some gas grills even come with a warming feature, which will keep your food warm while the rest of it finishes cooking.

Gas grills usually contain a built-in thermometer, which will aid you in cooking. You will know the exact temperature you are cooking at. Charcoal and Smoker grills do not typically contain this feature, which either leaves you guessing what temperatures you are cooking at or requires you to buy extra equipment to find out what temperature your food is.

Gas grills have safety concerns all of their own, but they are unmatched by other types of grills. Propane gas is highly flammable if not used correctly. Other grills, however, present higher opportunities for fire as they cook with an open flame. Gas grills are typically built much sturdier than their simpler counterparts.

If you are considering traveling with your barbeque grill, a gas grill may be the best option. Gas grills come in small sizes, which are perfect for traveling. Small-size gas containers are available at your local grocery store or department store, allowing you to transport the fuel source easily.

# HOW TO ELIMINATE OUTDOOR COOKING MISTAKES

We all make mistakes. When it comes to barbequing, this rule is the same. We often make mistakes that we do not even realize until we taste our food or something potentially dangerous happens.

Some mistakes mean that the food you cook will not taste delicious, while others could potentially mean a trip to the hospital or a visit from your claims representative on your home insurance policy. No matter the severity of the mistake, you should do your best to try to avoid them whenever possible.

## Most Common Cooking Mistakes

You must properly prepare the meat you are cooking before cooking it. It would be best if you never attempted to cook meat on a grill when it is still frozen or even partially frozen. Thaw your meat by sitting it out about 12 to 24 hours before you plan on cooking it or by thawing it in a microwave.

Once the meat is cooked, never put it back in on the same plate you had it on when it was raw; this could cause the spread of many unwanted illnesses.

Cooking with charcoal lighter fluid can be good or bad. The lighter fluid will cause the food you are cooking to taste different from other types of grills. Alternatively, attempting not to use lighter fluid may cause a lot of frustration because charcoal can be difficult, if not impossible, to light, without lighter fluid.

Never poke your meat while it is cooking. Poking holes in meat will cause the juice inside to leak out into the bottom of the grill. Not only will this make your food dry and unappealing in the end, but it also could potentially ruin your barbeque grill. At the very least, it will cause a buildup of unwanted grease and juices on your grill, which will make cleanup harder.

Once the meat is on the grill, try not to open the lid too many times. Each time you open the lid, you change the temperature in the grill. The constant change in temperature and the airflow will cause your meat to dry up quickly.

Remember that the higher the heat is not always, the better. While it is ok to quickly cook food, turning the heat up will cause the meat to dry up and potentially burn.

While using tin foil or aluminum foil will make cleaning easier, it will cause your food to have more of a fried taste than a grilled taste.

## Dangerous Mistakes

Never, under any circumstance, should you leave a grill alone when it is in use. Grilling does have fire involved, and accidents can happen. Fire spreads quickly, so being aware of your grill could mean the difference between a small fire that is quickly extinguished and a visit from the fire department.

Never place a hot grill against a wall, even if the fire is already completely out. A hot grill can heat an exterior wall to the point of combustion. Also, do not put the grill cover back on until you are sure that the grill is completely cool.

Your grill should be cleaned after every use, with no exceptions. While no one likes cleaning the grill, it is essential for your grill's life and safety. If you allow your grill to sit dirty, not only are you causing a potential fire and health hazard, but you are ultimately making it harder on yourself when it does come time to clean your grill.

Make sure that your grill is completely cold before cleaning it. Spraying oil and cleaning agents on a hot surface could cause it to ignite. Be careful because the grill may seem cool but may still be hot in certain areas. You do not want to sustain a burn.

# BBQ MAINTENANCE TIPS

When purchasing your barbeque grill, think of it as an investment rather than just another item for your outdoor entertainment. You should expect this item to become a large part of your outdoor activities for many years to come. But like any other investments, proper maintenance and care are needed to ensure that your barbeque grill will work for you for many years to come.

While some maintenance and cleaning are specific to the type of barbeque grill your own (gas, electric, charcoal, or smoke barbecue grill), the majority of care that should be carried on does not change from grill to grill.

## Step 1- Gathering the Necessary Items

You will need some everyday household items on hand when it comes time to clean your barbeque grill.

- Brass wire grill brush
- Steel wool pads, preferably that contain soap already.
- Mild dish soap
- Sponge or dishcloth
- Spray cooking oil
- Dry baking soda
- Aluminum foil

## Step 2- Brushing Your Grill Off

The first thing that should always be done to your grill is routine brushing. Using your brass wire grill brush (or other brush suitable to your type of grill), you should brush off all the surfaces. By routinely brushing your barbeque grill, you will prevent any buildup. If buildup from food is left too long, it can become increasingly difficult to remove.

## Step 3- Spray Cooking Oil

Once you are sure that your grill is free of all buildup and debris and that your grill is completely cooled off, you will want to spray it down with a light layer of cooking oil. Spraying it down with cooking oil will prevent your barbeque grill from rusting. It is essential to make sure your barbeque grill is completely cold, as spraying cooking oil on a hot surface may cause the oil to heat up and ignite, which could be potentially dangerous to you and your barbeque grill.

## Step 4- Use Baking Soda and Aluminum Foil on Your Grill

Baking soda is a very nice cleaning and polishing agent. Once you have removed any extra debris and buildup, lightly scrubbing your barbeque grill with baking soda will give it that extra shine, similar to when you brought it home from the store. This can also be used on handles and knobs to remove any additional buildup that cannot be taken off with a wire brush.

Aluminum foil can also be used to keep your grill looking nice. Gently rub the aluminum foil on your grill, and you will notice that it removes grim and buildup.

## Step 5- Clean Your Racks

The racks in your grill are important as this is where the food touches when it is cooking. You will have to use the wire brush to remove as much buildup as possible. Once you remove as much as possible, start washing the racks with dish soap. If the racks are dirty, you may also want to use steel wool pads. Be sure to completely rinse off all soap and residue before cooking on these racks again.

## Step 6- Preventing Problems

The majority of problems that arise from barbeque grills come from a lack of cleaning and maintenance. That means if you notice something does not seem quite right with your barbeque grill, chances are it can be fixed with just a simple cleaning. Even if you clean it and still find that it is having problems, at least you saved yourself the potential embarrassment of taking it to a professional only to find out all it needed was to be cleaned.

Finally, one method of preventing problems with your barbeque grill is protecting it from the outdoors. Covers are available for grills in all shapes and sizes, so chances are, you will find one that fits your grill. If you have a cover for your barbeque grill, then all you will ever need to do is do the regular maintenance listed above.

# SUMMER GRILLING

Summertime is the perfect time for barbequing. Not only are the temperatures perfect for outdoor activities, but often the children are out of school, and families are traveling for their summer vacations. Today in America, it is unheard of for a family to go an entire summer without having or attending a barbeque cookout. Today, over 90% of families attend a barbeque at least once a year.

Summer is indeed the perfect time to plan a barbeque party. It is essential to remember certain things when barbequing to ensure that your party goes flawless.

## Grilling Do's and Don'ts

1. Always start with a completely clean grill. The amazing fish you cooked last week was tasty, but unless you want a hint of fish with your hot dogs, you need to clean your grill before cooking. It is recommended that you clean your grill every time you use it. Please wait until it cools down, and then clean the surfaces with baking soda and the racks with grease-fighting dish soap and water.

2. Before you begin cooking, spray your cooking area with a nonstick cooking spray. This will prevent your meat from sticking when you are rotating or removing it. If your meat sticks and tears, you will lose a large amount of juice, and your meat may dry out.

3. Never place food on the grill until the temperature is correct. The fluctuation in temperatures will cause your food to dry out or burn. If you are using a charcoal grill, make sure that the coals are completely gray before putting the meat on the grill. This will allow the temperatures to level out and the majority of the lighter fluid to burn off.

4. While marinating before you cook will add flavor, covering your meat in barbeque sauces before cooking will dry your meat out and may even cause it to burn. This happens because most barbeque sauces contain high amounts of fat and sugar, which burn easily. Alternatively, lightly seasoning your meat will work well and will not have any adverse effects. If you must use barbeque sauce, only add it in the final minutes before taking your meat off the grill. Just remember that meat has a natural flavor that is only brought out by barbequing, so you do not want to ruin that.

5. Searing your meat will lock in the juices and taste, but you do not want to cook your meat at that temperature for the whole amount of time. Once you have seared both sides, reduce the heat to medium. This will ensure that your meat is full of flavor and tender.

6. Once the meat is cooked, never put it back in on the same plate you had when it was raw. This could cause the spread of many unwanted illnesses. Do not handle cooked meat with the same utensils that you used when it was raw.

7. Never poke your meat while it is cooking. Poking holes in meat will cause the juice inside to leak out into the bottom of the grill. Not only will this make your food dry and unappealing in the end, but it also could potentially ruin your barbeque grill. At the very least, it will cause a buildup of unwanted grease and juices on your grill, which will make cleanup harder.

# 1 – Kebabs BBQ Salmon

| Preparation | Cooking | Servings |
|:---:|:---:|:---:|
| 20 min | 10 min | 6 |

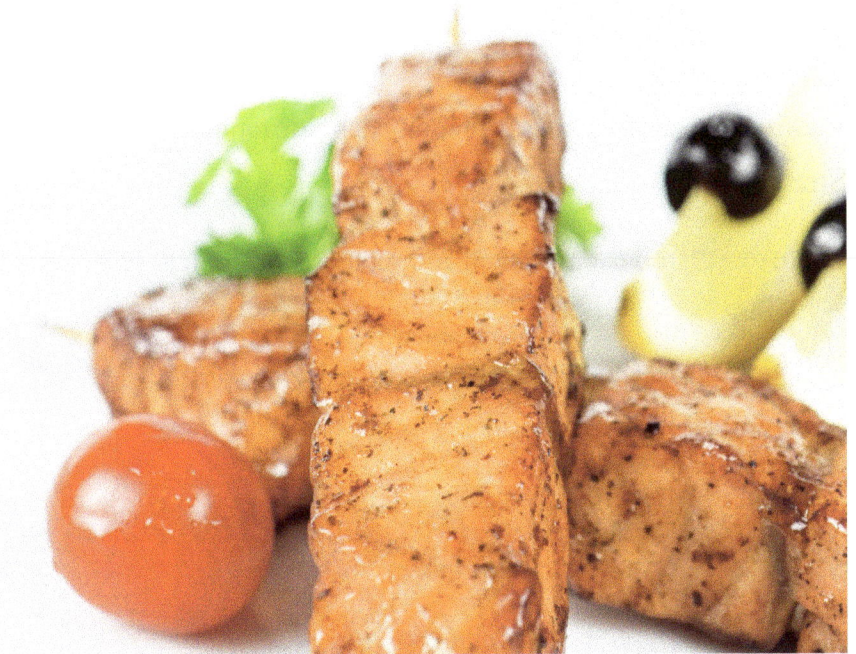

## Ingredients:

- 2 shallots, ends trimmed, halved
- 3 zucchinis, cut in 2-inch cubes
- 2 cup cherry tomatoes
- 6 skinless salmon fillets, cut into 1-inch pieces

- 4 limes, cut into thin wedges

## Directions:

### Step 1
Preheat a barbecue or char grill on medium-high.
Thread fish cubes onto skewers, then zucchinis, shallots and tomatoes.

### Step 2
Repeat to make 12 kebabs.
Bake the kebabs for about 3 minutes each side for medium cooked.

### Step 3

Move to a plate, cover with foil and set aside for 5 min to rest before serving.

**Nutrition: Calories: 350  Carbs: 9g  Fat: 19g  Protein: 40 g**

# 2 - Lemon Fish Fillets

| Preparation | Cooking | Servings |
| --- | --- | --- |
| 15 min | 15 min | 4 |

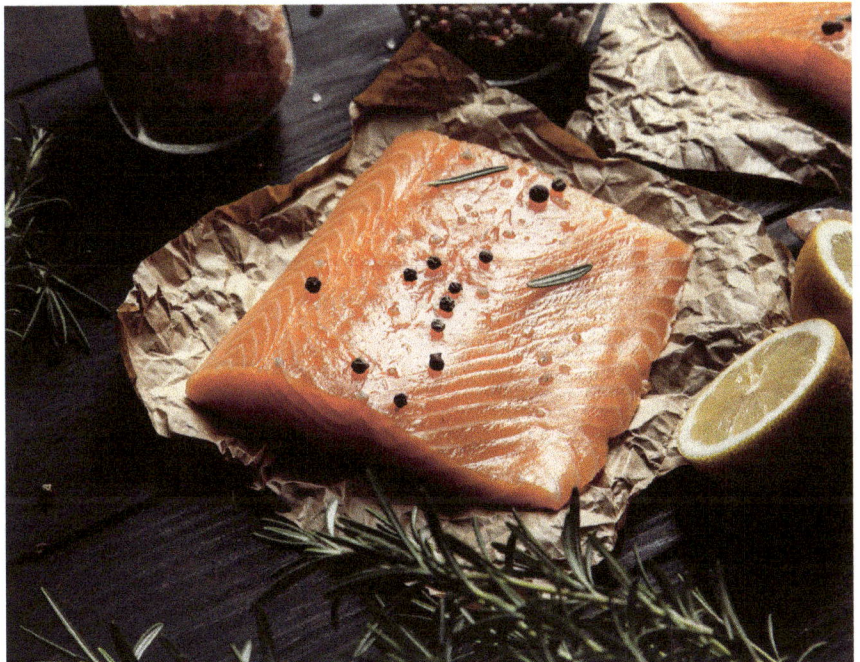

## Ingredients:

- 4 white fish fillets
- 2 tbsp dried rosemary
- 5 tbsp breadcrumbs
- 3 tbsp lemon zest

- 1 tsp garlic powder

- 3 tbsp extra virgin olive oil

- 1 tsp salt

## Directions:

### Step 1
Combine the rosemary, breadcrumbs, lemon zest, garlic powder and salt in a food processor and blend until well mixed.

### Step 2
Add the fish fillets, skin-side up, on a lined baking tray.
Grill for 3-4 minutes.

### Step 3
Turn the fish over and press a quarter of the breadcrumb mixture over the top of each fillet.

### Step 4
Drizzle with olive oil and grill for 4 min until the crust is golden and the fish is cooked through.

Serve with steamed spinach or baked potatoes.

**Nutrition: Calories: 90 Carbs: 10g Fat: 8g Protein: 31g**

# 3 - Thay Salmon with Broccoli

| Preparation | Cooking | Servings |
|:---:|:---:|:---:|
| 15 min | 15 min | 4 |

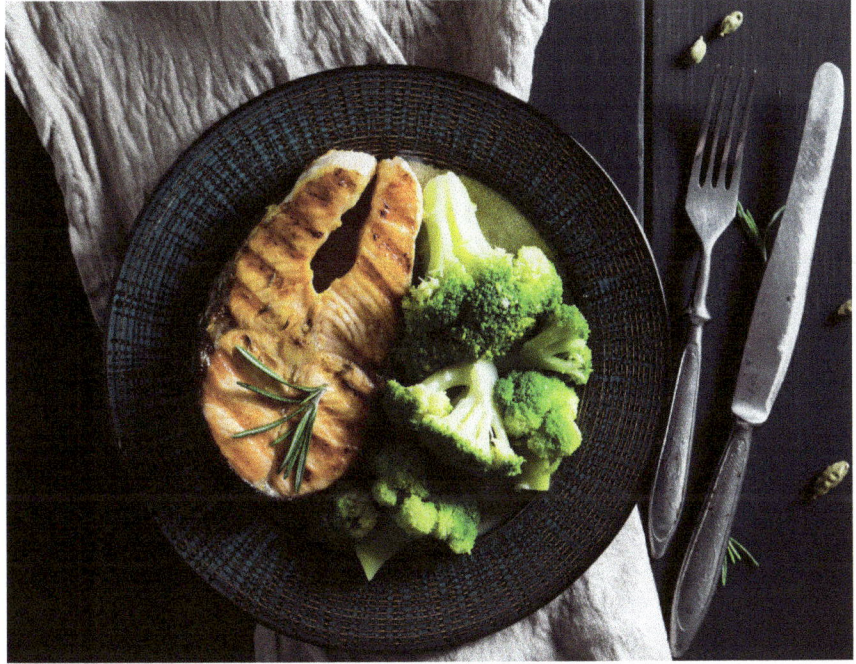

## Ingredients:

- 4 salmon fillets, skin on
- 1 lb. fresh broccoli florets
- 3 tbsp soy sauce
- 3 tbsp toasted sesame oil

- 2 tsp chili garlic sauce

- 1 tbsp brown sugar

- 1 cup green onions, finely cut, to serve

## Directions:

### Step 1
Combine the garlic and soy sauce with the sesame oil and brown sugar in a large bowl.
### Step 2
Add in the salmon and broccoli and toss to coat.
Place salmon skin side down in a single layer on a lined baking tray.
### Step 3
Add the broccoli florets around.
Bake 10-12 minutes or until the fish is cooked through and flakes easily with a fork.
### Step 4

Top with green onions and serve.

**Nutrition: Calories: 356 Carbs: 11g Fat: 19g Protein: 27g**

# 4 - BBQ Salmon with Spinach

| Preparation | Cooking | Servings |
|:---:|:---:|:---:|
| 15 min | 10 min | 4 |

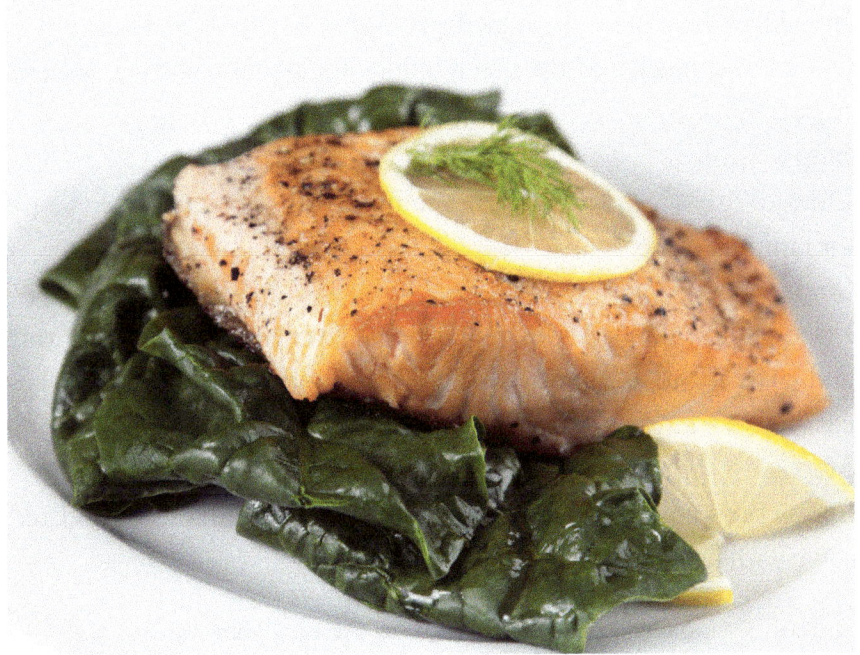

## Ingredients:

- 4 salmon fillets, skin on
- 2 bag frozen spinach
- 5 green onions, chopped
- 2 cup crumbled feta cheese

- 5 tbsp extra virgin olive oil

- Salt and pepper, to taste

- Lemon wedges, to serve

## Directions:

### Step 1
In a skillet, heat olive oil on medium-high.
Cook the spinach and the green onions for 2-3 min, stirring once or twice.

### Step 2
Drizzle with salt and pepper to taste and add in the feta cheese. Cook for 1 minute more.

### Step 3
Place salmon skin side down in a single layer on a lined baking tray and roast for 10-12 minutes or until it is cooked through and flakes easily with a fork.

### Step 4
Spoon the spinach mixture onto plates, then top with the salmon and serve with lemon wedges.

**Nutrition: Calories: 350 Carbs: 6g Fat: 15g Protein: 21g**

# 5 - BBQ Shrimp

| Preparation | Cooking | Servings |
|:---:|:---:|:---:|
| 25 min | 25 min | 4 |

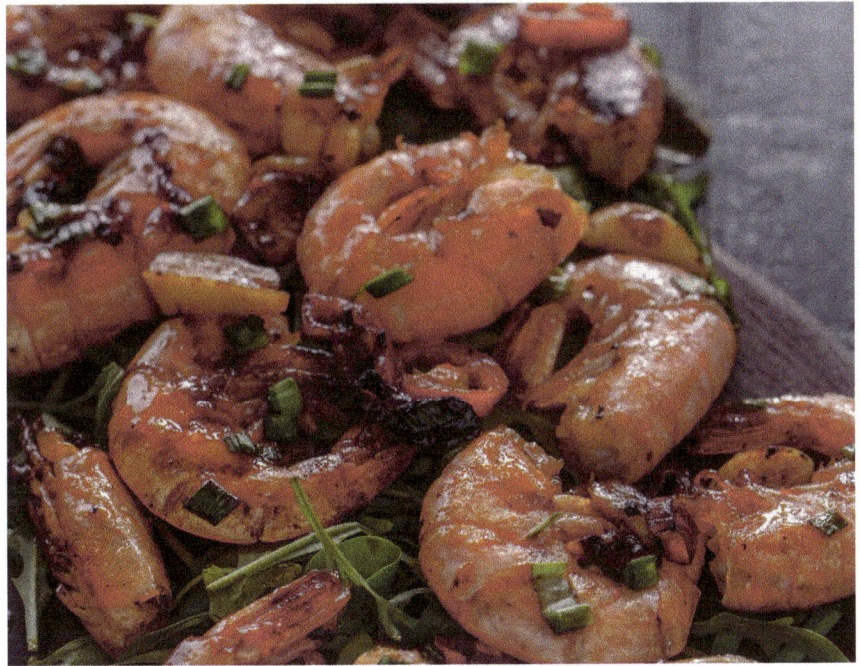

## Ingredients:

- 6 tablespoons olive oil, divided
- 1 yellow onion, diced small
- 3 cups grits
- 6 cups water

- 1 cup shredded Cheddar cheese

- 2 teaspoons salt

- 1 teaspoon ground black pepper

- 2 pounds shrimp, peeled and deveined

- 1 teaspoon smoked paprika

- 2 teaspoons ground cumin

- 1 cup vinegar-based Carolina-style BBQ sauce

## Directions:

### Step 1

Preheat the grill to high heat.

### Step 2

Heat 1 tablespoon of olive oil in a large pot on medium-high heat. Add the onions and brown, about 6 to 8 minutes. Add in the grits and 6 cups of water and stir over medium-low heat until the grits have absorbed the water and are cooked through, about 20 to 25 minutes. Whisk the cheese into the grits and season with salt and pepper. Keep warm.

### Step 3

Line a hot grill with Reynolds Wrap® Heavy Duty Aluminum Foil.

### Step 4

Combine the shrimp, paprika, cumin, and remaining 3 tablespoons of olive oil in a bowl and mix.

## Step 5

Place the shrimp right onto the foil on the grill and cook for 3 to 4 minutes on each side or until browned and cooked throughout.

## Step 6

Pour the BBQ sauce on top of the shrimp and mix.

## Step 7

Serve shrimp with the cheesy grits.

Per Serving: 922 calories; protein 70.4g; carbohydrates 88.1g; fat 36.1g; cholesterol 394.7mg; sodium 2928.8mg.

# 6 – BBQ Chili Shrimp

| Preparation | Cooking | Servings |
|:---:|:---:|:---:|
| 20 min | 10 min | 4 |

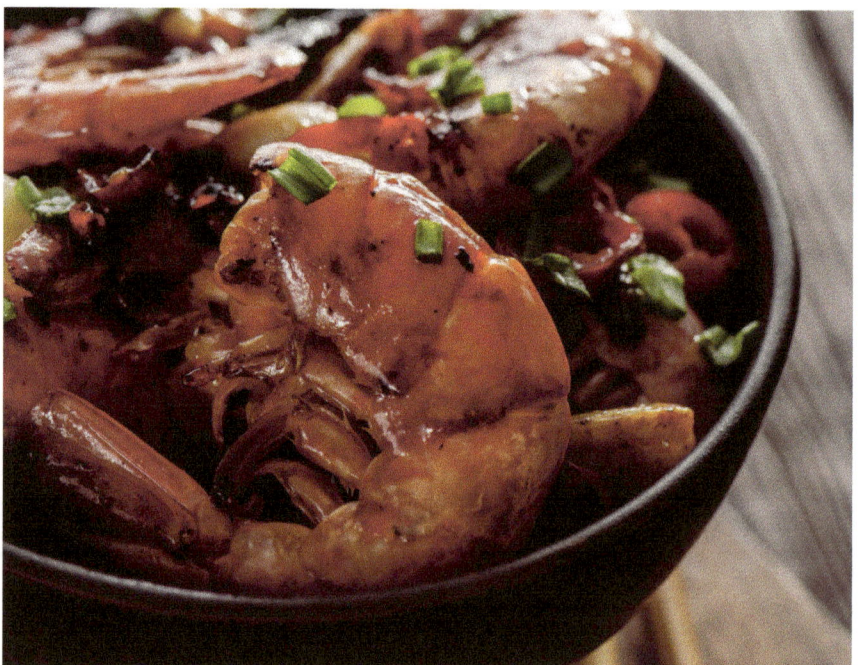

## Ingredients:

- 1 pound extra large shrimp (16-20 per lb.), shell on, deveined
- 1 teaspoon salt
- $\frac{1}{4}$ teaspoon black pepper
- 1 tablespoon brown sugar

- 2 tablespoon lemon juice
- 1 tablespoon ketchup
- 2 teaspoon chili powder
- 1 teaspoon ground cumin
- $\frac{1}{4}$ teaspoon ground allspice
- $\frac{1}{4}$ teaspoon cayenne pepper
- 2 tablespoon vegetable oil
- Lemon wedges

## Directions:

### Step 1

Season with salt, pepper, brown sugar, chili powder, cumin, allspice, cayenne pepper, lemon juice, ketchup. Pour in olive oil and stir thoroughly. Let shrimp sit for about 15 minutes, no longer.

### Step 2

Heat a dry saute pan over medium-high heat until hot but not smoking, or when a few drops of water sizzle and start to bead up before evaporating. Place shrimp in pan. Let cook on one side until the shrimp turns from opaque to white about halfway up the side, 3 or 4 minutes. Turn shrimp over. Cook until shrimp are almost cooked through. Transfer to a serving plate.

Per Serving: 192 calories; protein 19.9g; carbohydrates 8g; fat 6.7g; cholesterol 192.6mg; sodium 985mg.

# 7 - BBQ Shrimp with Citrus

| Preparation | Cooking | Servings |
|:---:|:---:|:---:|
| 25 min | 25 min | 4 |

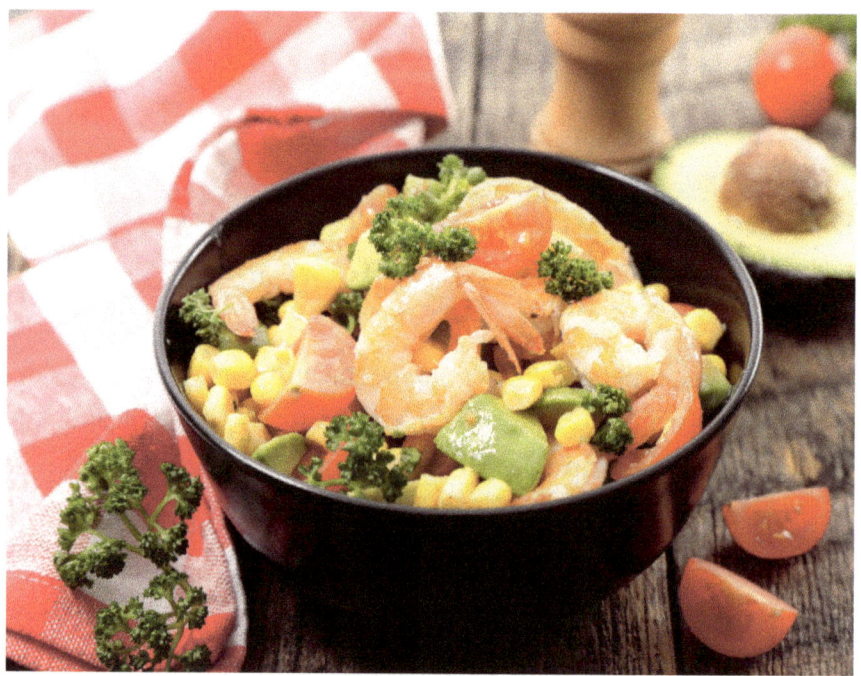

## Ingredients:

- 15 each large or jumbo raw shrimp, peeled and deveined (tails left on)
- $\frac{1}{4}$ cup finely chopped fresh cilantro
- 4 tablespoons lime juice

- 1 teaspoon ground black pepper, or more to taste
- 1 teaspoon sea salt, or more to taste
- 2tablespoons barbeque sauce, or more as desired
- 1 sheet Heavy Duty Aluminum Foil

## Citrus Corn Salad:

- 1 (16 ounce) package frozen corn
- 1 cup chopped fresh cilantro
- 1 cup thinly sliced celery
- 1 cup diced red bell pepper
- $\frac{1}{4}$ cup diced red onion
- 1 cup halved grape tomatoes
- 3 tablespoons lime juice, or more to taste
- 1 teaspoon apple cider vinegar, or more to taste
- 1 teaspoon sea salt, or more to taste
- 2 teaspoon ground black pepper, or more to taste

## Directions:

### Step 1
Set grill to medium heat.
### Step 2
Clean and remove shell from shrimp (leaving tail on).
### Step 3
In plastic container or bag add shrimp, cilantro, lime juice, ground black pepper and sea salt, place in refrigerator and allow to marinate for minimum of 30 minutes (overnight will give the best flavor).

### Step 4

Place marinated shrimp on sheet of Heavy-Duty Foil, pour BBQ sauce over shrimp, fold aluminum foil up and fold over twice; fold each end. Leave enough room for air to circulate in packet.

### Step 5

Place packet on grill and allow to cook 6 to 8 minutes.

### Step 6

Citrus Corn Salad: In a large skillet over medium heat add corn and granulated sugar, allow to cook 8 to 10 minutes.

### Step 7

Add ice and water to large bowl to make ice bath and pour corn into ice bath, drain in colander, pour corn back into the bowl and add the cilantro, celery, red pepper, red onion, grape tomatoes, lime juice, apple cider vinegar, sea salt and ground black pepper and mix together to incorporate.

Per Serving: 252 calories; protein 14.7g; carbohydrates 38.2g; fat 4.3g; cholesterol 78mg; sodium 852.5mg.

# 8 - BBQ Shrimp Garlic Marinade

| Preparation | Cooking | Servings |
|:---:|:---:|:---:|
| 25 min | 35 min | 4 |

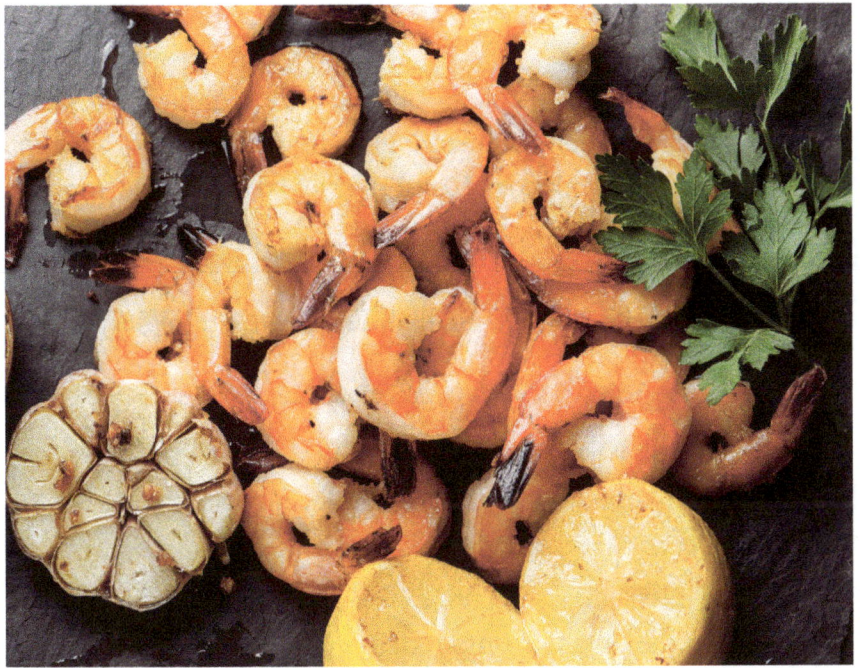

## Ingredients:

- 2 cup canola oil

- 1 teaspoon hot pepper sauce (such as Tabasco®)

- 3 cloves garlic, crushed

- 1 cup tomato-based chili sauce

- 1 lemon, juiced

- 1 teaspoon dried oregano

- 2 pounds peeled and deveined medium shrimp

- 16 skewers

## Directions:

### Step 1
Whisk together the canola oil, hot pepper sauce, garlic, chili sauce, lemon juice, and oregano in a large glass or ceramic bowl. Add the shrimp and toss to evenly coat. Cover the bowl with plastic wrap, and marinate in the refrigerator 1 hour.

### Step 2
Preheat an outdoor grill for medium-high heat, and lightly oil the grate.

### Step 3
Remove the shrimp from the marinade, and shake off excess. Discard the remaining marinade. Thread about 4 shrimp onto each skewer.

### Step 4
Cook on the preheated grill until pink on the outside and no longer translucent in the center, about 3 minutes per side.

Per Serving: 125 calories; protein 19g; carbohydrates 3.9g; fat 3.8g; cholesterol 172.8mg; sodium 324.7mg.

# 9 - BBQ Fish Fillet with Pesto Sauce

| Preparation | Cooking | Servings |
|:---:|:---:|:---:|
| 10 min | 15 min | 4 |

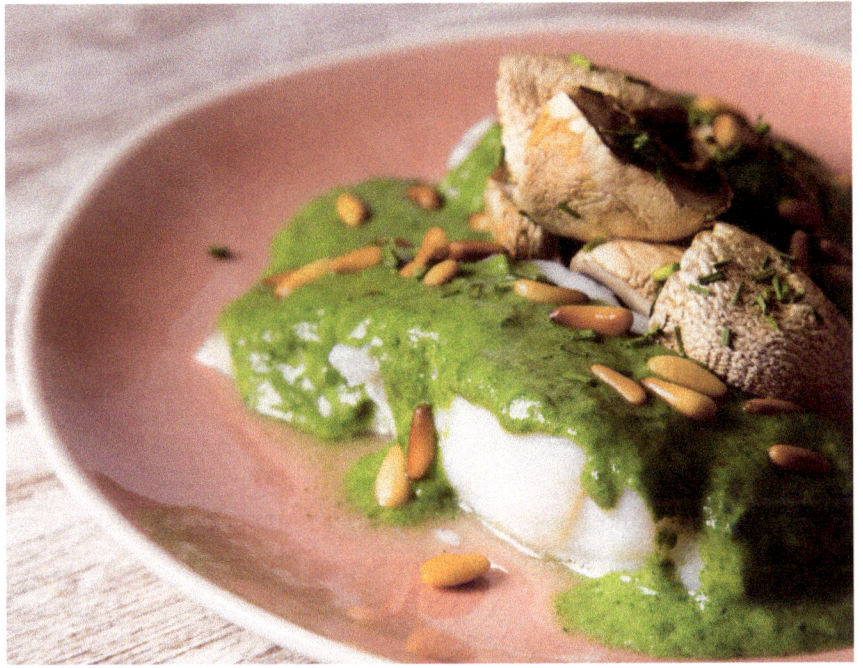

## Ingredients:

- 4 white fish fillets (200 g each)
- 2 tablespoon olive oil
- pepper & sal

## Pesto Sauce:

- 2 bunch fresh basil
- 4 garlic cloves
- 2 tablespoon pine nuts
- 1 tablespoon grated Parmesan cheese
- 2 cup extra-virgin olive oil
- $\frac{1}{2}$ pound mushrooms (optional)

## Directions:

### Step 1

Heat the Philips Airfryer to 180C. Brush the fish fillets with the oil and season with pepper & salt.

### Step 2

Place in the cooking basket of the Airfryer and slide the basket into the Philips Airfryer. Set the timer for 8 minutes.

### Step 3

Pick the basil leaves and place them with the garlic, pine nuts, Parmesan cheese and olive oil in a food processor or pestle and mortar.

### Step 4

Pulse or grind the mixture until it turns into a sauce. Add some salt to taste.

## Step 5

Place the fish fillets with mushrooms on a serving plate and serve them drizzled with the pesto sauce.

Nutrition: 1142 calories; protein 53.7g; carbohydrates 4.1g; fat 223.5g; cholesterol 65.3mg; sodium 1477.2mg.

# 10 - Alaskan BBQ Salmon

| Preparation | Cooking | Servings |
|:---:|:---:|:---:|
| 15 min | 15 min | 8 |

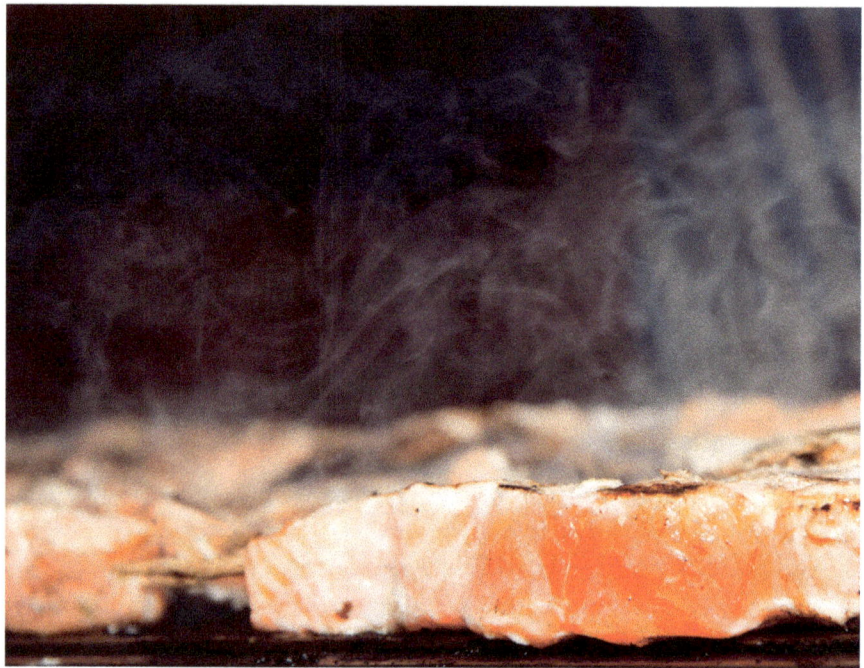

## Ingredients:

- 1 cup brown sugar
- $\frac{1}{2}$ cup honey
- 1 dash liquid smoke flavoring
- $\frac{1}{2}$ cup apple cider vinegar

- 1 (4 pound) whole salmon fillet

## Directions:

### Step 1
Preheat grill for high heat.

### Step 2
In a small bowl, mix together brown sugar, honey, liquid smoke, and vinegar.

### Step 3
Brush one side of the salmon with the basting sauce. Place the salmon on the grill, basted side down. After about 7 minutes, generously baste the top, and turn over. Cook for about 8 more minutes, then brush on more basting sauce, turn, and cook for 2 minutes. Take care not to overcook the salmon as it will lose its juices and flavor if cooked too long.

Per Serving: 269 calories; protein 19.6g; carbohydrates 22.3g; fat 11g; cholesterol 55.9mg; sodium 58.7mg.

# II - BBQ Salmon in Butter Sauce

| Preparation | Cooking | Servings |
|:---:|:---:|:---:|
| 10 min | 20 min | 4 |

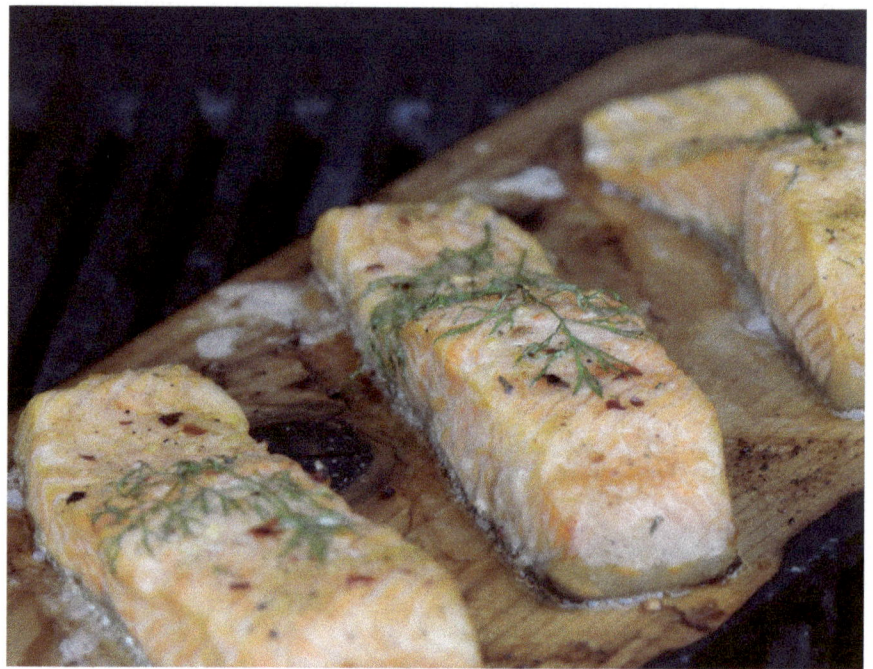

## Ingredients:

- ⅓ cup butter
- ½ small onion, or to taste, diced
- 1 teaspoon Worcestershire sauce
- ¼ teaspoon paprika

- 4 salmon steaks

## Directions:

### Step 1

Preheat grill for medium heat.

### Step 2

Melt butter in a saucepan; stir onion, Worcestershire sauce, and paprika into the melted butter.

### Step 3

Arrange four squares of aluminum foil on a flat work surface. Place a salmon steak in the middle of each piece of foil. Roll edges toward the salmon to make miniature pans and pour about 1/4 of the butter sauce over each steak.

### Step 4

Carefully set 'pans' onto the hot grill and cook until the fish flakes easily with a fork, 20 to 25 minutes.

Per Serving: 427 calories; protein 36.5g; carbohydrates 1.2g; fat 29.9g; cholesterol 156.2mg; sodium 210.9mg.

# 12 - Blueberry-BBQ Salmon

| Preparation | Cooking | Servings |
|:---:|:---:|:---:|
| 5 min | 5 min | 4 |

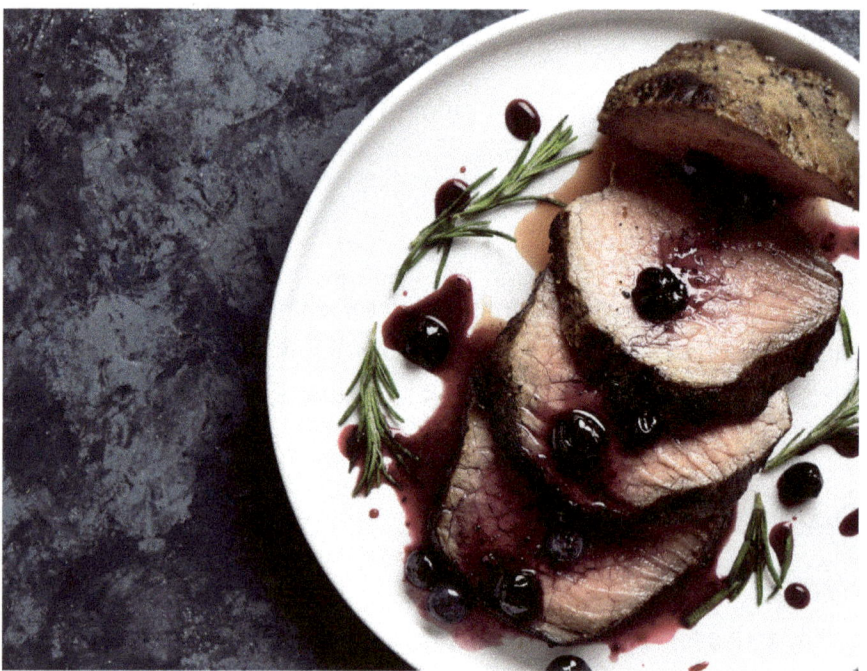

## Ingredients:

- 2 tablespoons barbeque sauce

- 2 teaspoons blueberry jam

- 1 (1 pound) fillet salmon

## Directions:

### Step 1
Set an oven rack about 6 inches from the heat source and preheat the oven's broiler. Line a baking sheet with parchment paper.

### Step 2
Mix together barbecue sauce and blueberry jam in a small bowl until well combined. Place salmon on the prepared baking sheet and cover with 2/3 of the sauce. Reserve remaining sauce.

### Step 3
Broil the salmon in the preheated oven until fish flakes easily with a fork, 5 to 10 minutes. Remove from the oven and cover with the remaining sauce to serve.

Per Serving: 184 calories; protein 24.2g; carbohydrates 5.1g; fat 6.7g; cholesterol 50.4mg; sodium 135.4mg.

# 13 - Chile Garlic BBQ Salmon

| Preparation | Cooking | Servings |
|:---:|:---:|:---:|
| 15 min | 35 min | 4 |

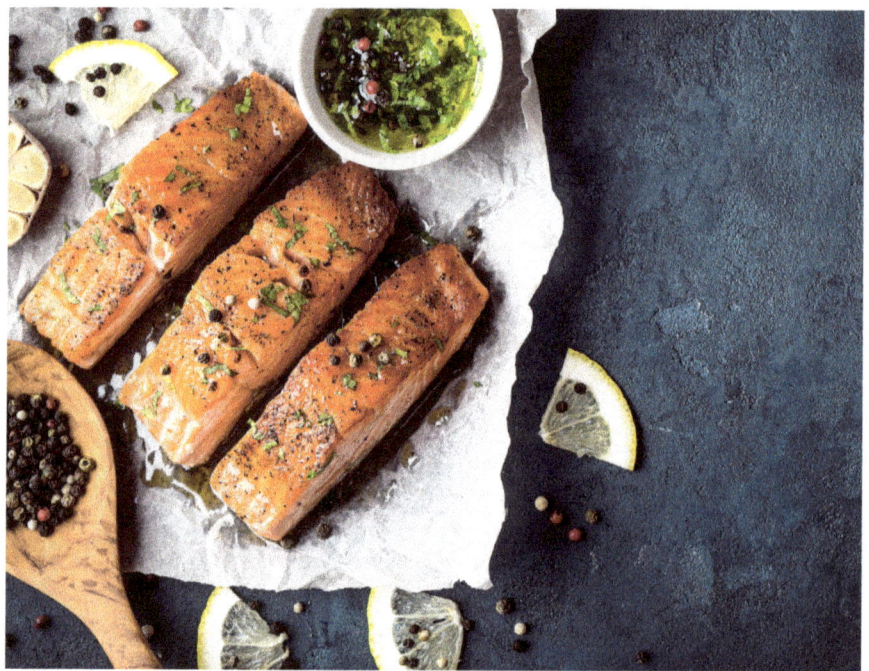

## Ingredient:

- 3 pounds whole salmon, cleaned
- $\frac{1}{4}$ cup soy sauce
- 1 tablespoon chile sauce
- 1 tablespoon chopped fresh ginger root

- 1 clove garlic, chopped
- 1 lime, juiced
- 1 lime, zested
- 1 tablespoon brown sugar
- 3 green onions, chopped

## Directions:

### Step 1

Prepare outdoor grill for high heat.

### Step 2

Trim the tail and fins off of the salmon. Make several shallow cuts across the salmon's skin. Place salmon on 3 larges, slightly overlapping sheets of aluminum foil.

### Step 3

In a bowl, stir together soy sauce, chile sauce, ginger, and garlic. Mix in lime juice, lime zest, and brown sugar. Spoon sauce over the salmon.

### Step 4

Fold the foil over the salmon, and crimp the edges to seal.

### Step 5

If using hot coals, move them to one side of the grill. Place the fish on the side of the grill that does not have coals directly underneath it, and close the lid. If using a gas grill, place the fish on one side, and turn off the flames directly underneath it; close the lid. Cook for 25 to 30 minutes. Remove to a serving platter, and pour any juices that may have collected in the foil over the top of the fish. Sprinkle with green onions.

Per Serving: 438 calories; protein 46.2g; carbohydrates 5.3g; fat 24.7g; cholesterol 133.9mg; sodium 737.5mg.

# 14 - Firecracker Grilled Alaska Salmon

| Preparation | Cooking | Servings |
|:---:|:---:|:---:|
| 20 min | 20 min | 8 |

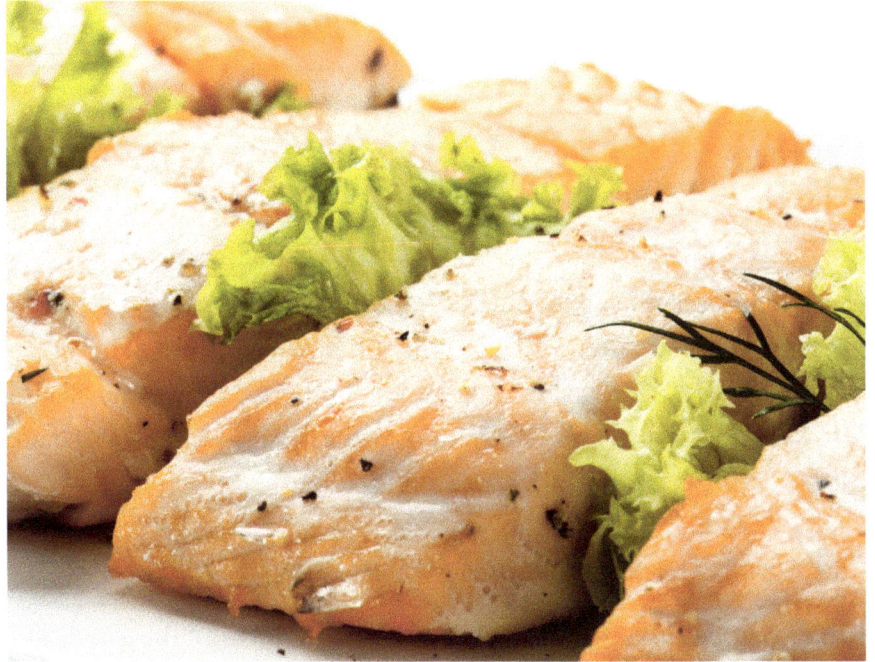

## Ingredients:

- 8 (4 ounce) fillets salmon
- ½ cup peanut oil
- 4 tablespoons soy sauce
- 4 tablespoons balsamic vinegar

- 4 tablespoons green onions, chopped

- 3 teaspoons brown sugar

- 2 cloves garlic, minced

- 1 ½ teaspoons ground ginger

- 2 teaspoons crushed red pepper flakes

- 1 teaspoon sesame oil

- ½ teaspoon salt

## Directions:

### Step 1

Place salmon filets in a medium, nonporous glass dish. In a separate medium bowl, combine the peanut oil, soy sauce, vinegar, green onions, brown sugar, garlic, ginger, red pepper flakes, sesame oil and salt. Whisk together well, and pour over the fish. Cover and marinate the fish in the refrigerator for 4 to 6 hours.

### Step 2

Prepare an outdoor grill with coals about 5 inches from the grate, and lightly oil the grate.

### Step 3

Grill the fillets 5 inches from coals for 10 minutes per inch of thickness, measured at the thickest part, or until fish just flakes with a fork. Turn over halfway through cooking.

Per Serving: 307 calories; protein 23.3g; carbohydrates 4.6g; fat 21.5g; cholesterol 62.9mg; sodium 649.3mg.

# 15 - Grilled Tilapia with Smoked Paprika

| Preparation | Cooking | Servings |
|:---:|:---:|:---:|
| 15 min | 15 min | 4 |

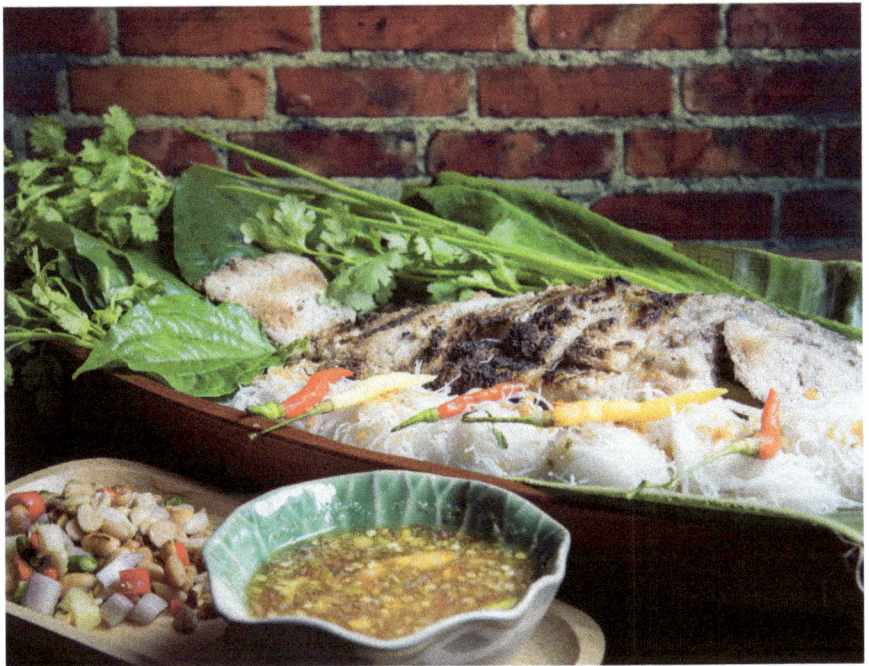

## Ingredients:

- 3 tablespoons olive oil
- 2 teaspoons ground smoked paprika
- 1 teaspoon garlic powder
- $\frac{1}{2}$ teaspoon salt

- $\frac{1}{2}$ teaspoon freshly ground black pepper
- 4 (6 ounce) tilapia fillets
- cooking spray

## Directions:

## Step 1

Combine olive oil, paprika, garlic powder, salt, and black pepper in a small bowl; stir well. Brush oil mixture evenly over tilapia fillets.

## Step 2

Heat a large nonstick grill pan over medium-high heat; grease with cooking spray. Grill fish until it flakes easily with a fork, about 4 minutes per side.

Per Serving: 264 calories; protein 34.8g; carbohydrates 1.3g; fat 12.5g; cholesterol 61.6mg; sodium 367.2mg.

# 16 - Grilled Tuna Steaks with Grape and Caper Salsa

| Preparation | Cooking | Servings |
|:---:|:---:|:---:|
| 20 min | 10 min | 4 |

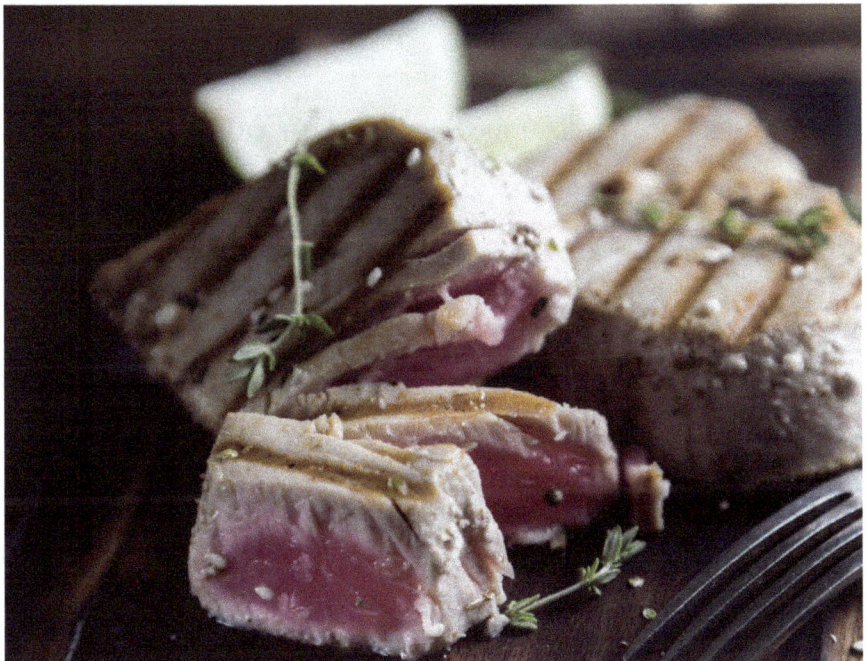

## Ingredients:

- 2 cups red seedless grapes, halved
- ⅓ cup capers, drained and rinsed
- 1 shallot, minced
- 2 tablespoons chopped fresh parsley

- 1 tablespoon olive oil

- salt and black pepper to taste

- 4 (8 ounce) tuna steaks

- $\frac{1}{4}$ cup fresh lemon juice

## Directions:

### Step 1

Preheat an outdoor grill for medium-high heat and lightly oil grate.

### Step 2

Stir together grapes, capers, shallot, parsley, and olive oil in a bowl; season to taste with salt and pepper, and set aside. Place tuna steaks onto a plate, and brush with lemon juice. Season with salt and pepper to taste.

### Step 3

Cook tuna steaks on preheated grill until cooked to desired degree of doneness, 2 to 3 minutes per side for medium-rare. Serve with the grape and caper salsa.

Per Serving: 348 calories; protein 54.1g; carbohydrates 18.3g; fat 6.1g; cholesterol 102.4mg; sodium 427.2mg.

# 17 - Spicy Grilled Shrimp

| Preparation | Cooking | Servings |
|:---:|:---:|:---:|
| 45 min | 5 min | 4 |

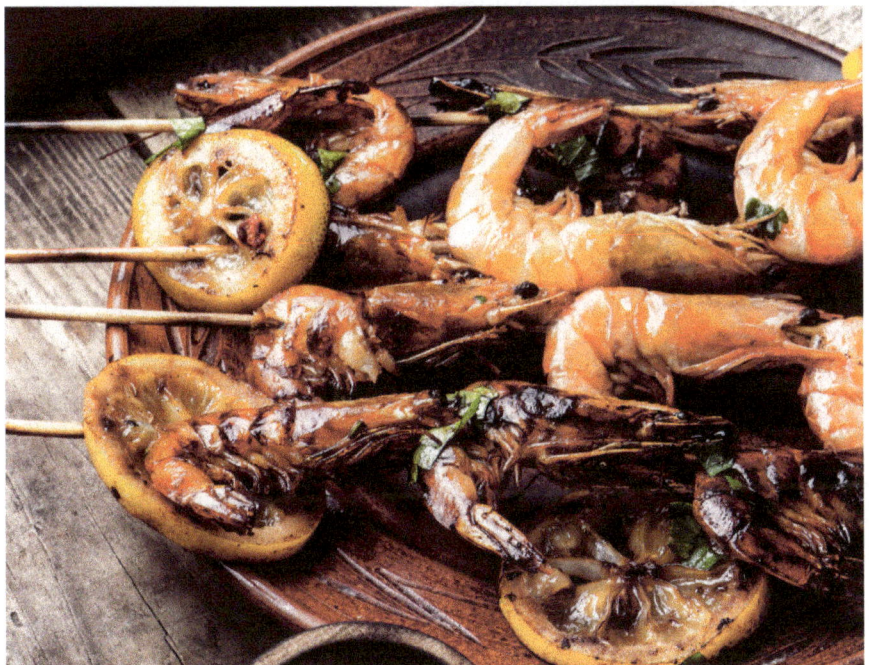

## Ingredients:

- ⅓ cup olive oil
- ¼ cup sesame oil
- ¼ cup chopped fresh parsley
- 2 tablespoons hot sauce

- 2 tablespoons minced garlic

- 1 tablespoon ketchup

- 1 tablespoon Asian chile paste

- 1 teaspoon salt

- 1 teaspoon black pepper

- 3 tablespoons lemon juice

- 2 pounds large shrimp, peeled and deveined

- 12 wooden skewers, soaked in water

### Directions:

### Step 1

Whisk together the olive oil, sesame oil, parsley, hot sauce, minced garlic, ketchup, chile sauce, salt, pepper, and lemon juice in a mixing bowl. Set aside about 1/3 of this marinade to use while grilling.

### Step 2

Place the shrimp in a large, resealable plastic bag. Pour in the remaining marinade and seal the bag. Refrigerate for 2 hours.

### Step 3

Preheat an outdoor grill for high heat. Thread shrimp onto skewers, piercing once near the tail and once near the head. Discard marinade.

### Step 4

Lightly oil grill grate. Cook shrimp for 2 minutes per side until opaque, basting frequently with reserved marinade.

Per Serving: 320 calories; protein 25.1g; carbohydrates 4.1g; fat 22.8g; cholesterol 230.4mg; sodium 827.3mg.

# 18 - Grilled Spicy Shrimp Tacos

| Preparation | Cooking | Servings |
| --- | --- | --- |
| 15 min | 25 min | 6 |

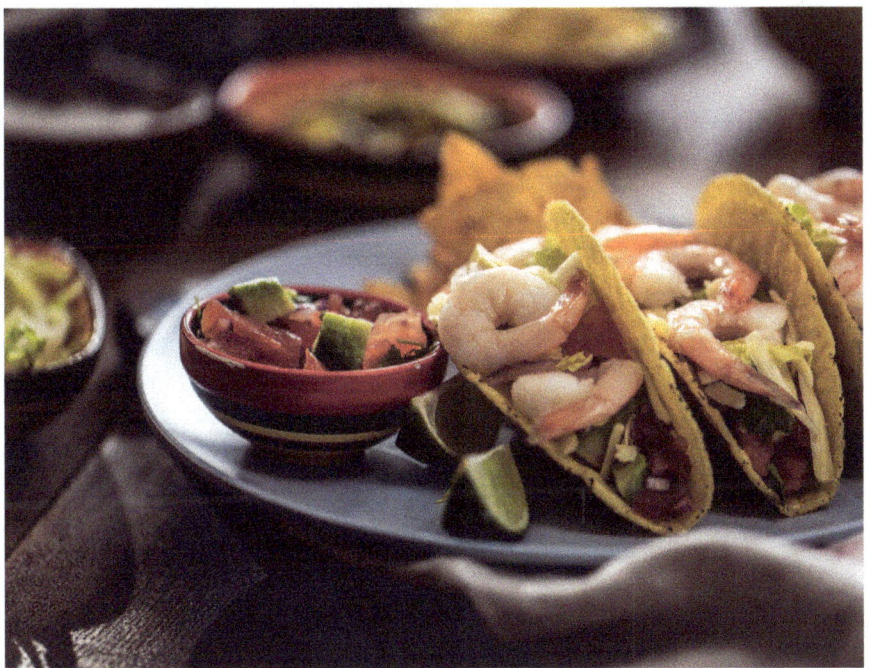

## Ingredients:

## Shrimp Marinade:

- 1 ½ cups lime juice
- 3 tablespoons olive oil
- 2 tablespoons chili powder

- 1 teaspoon mayonnaise

- 3 pounds uncooked medium shrimp, peeled and deveined

## Chipotle Sauce:

- $\frac{1}{2}$ cup enchilada sauce

- $\frac{1}{2}$ (4 ounce) jar diced jalapeno peppers

- 5 teaspoons honey

- 3 teaspoons lime juice

- salt to taste

## Red Slaw:

$\frac{1}{2}$ head red cabbage, shredded, or more to taste

2 bunches scallions, chopped

3 tablespoons olive oil

3 tablespoons white vinegar

1 small bunch cilantro, chopped

20 (8 inch) corn tortillas

## Directions:

### Step 1

Mix lime juice, olive oil, chili powder, and mayonnaise together in a bowl. Add shrimp and marinade for at least 1 hour.

### Step 2

Mix enchilada sauce, jalapenos, honey, lime juice, and salt together in a separate bowl for the sauce.

### Step 3

Toss cabbage with scallions, olive oil, vinegar, and cilantro in a large bowl for the slaw.

### Step 4

Heat tortillas in a frying pan over medium-high heat, about 30 seconds per side. Keep warm.

### Step 5

Preheat an outdoor grill for medium heat and lightly oil the grate.

### Step 6

Remove shrimp from marinade. Grill until opaque, about 5 minutes. Add shrimp to each tortilla; top with the sauce and slaw.

**Per Serving: 187 calories; protein 13.9g; carbohydrates 20.9g; fat 6.1g; cholesterol 103.7mg; sodium 226.1mg.**

## 19 - Grilled Tequila-Lime Shrimp

| Preparation | Cooking | Servings |
|:---:|:---:|:---:|
| 10 min | 6 min | 4 |

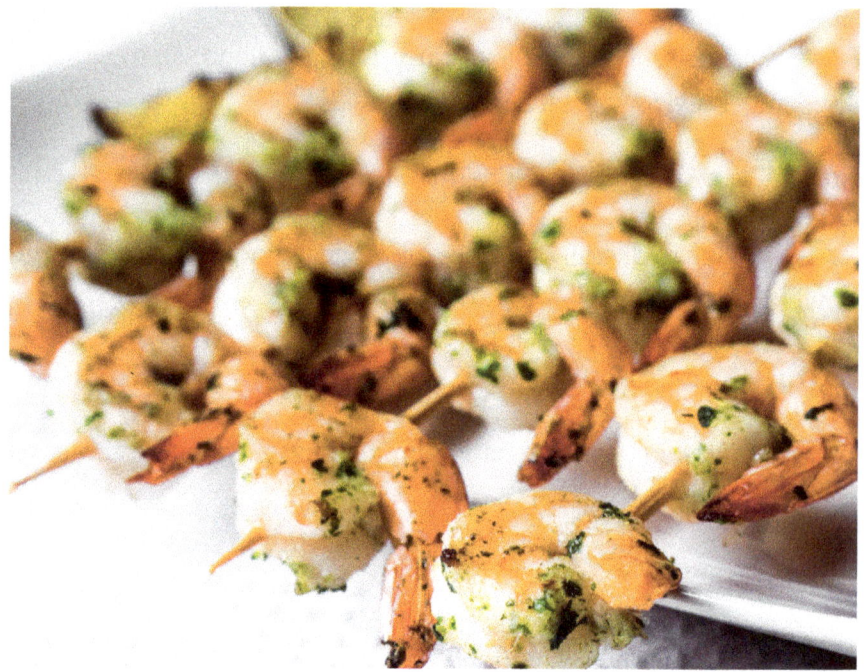

## Ingredient:

- 2 tablespoons lime juice
- 2 tablespoons tequila
- $\frac{1}{4}$ cup olive oil
- 1 pinch garlic salt

- 1 pinch ground cumin
- ground black pepper to taste
- 1-pound large shrimp, peeled and deveined
- 6 (10 inch) wooden skewers
- 1 large lime, quartered

## Directions:

### Step 1

Whisk together the lime juice, tequila, olive oil, garlic salt, cumin, and black pepper in a bowl until well blended. Pour into a large resealable plastic bag; add the shrimp, seal bag

and turn to coat evenly. Refrigerate 1 to 4 hours before grilling.

### Step 2

Soak skewers at least 30 minutes in water to prevent burning.

### Step 3

Preheat outdoor grill for medium-high heat. Lightly oil grill grate, and place about 4 inches from heat source.

### Step 4

Drain and discard marinade from shrimp. Thread shrimp onto prepared skewers, 5 to 6 per skewer.

## Step 5

Cook, uncovered, on preheated grill until shrimp turn pink, turning once, for 5 to 7 minutes. Serve with lime wedges for garnish.

Per Serving: 235 calories; protein 18.8g; carbohydrates 3.8g; fat 14.6g; cholesterol 172.9mg; sodium 282.5mg.

# 20 - Grilled Salmon

| Preparation | Cooking | Servings |
|:---:|:---:|:---:|
| 10 min | 10 min | 4 |

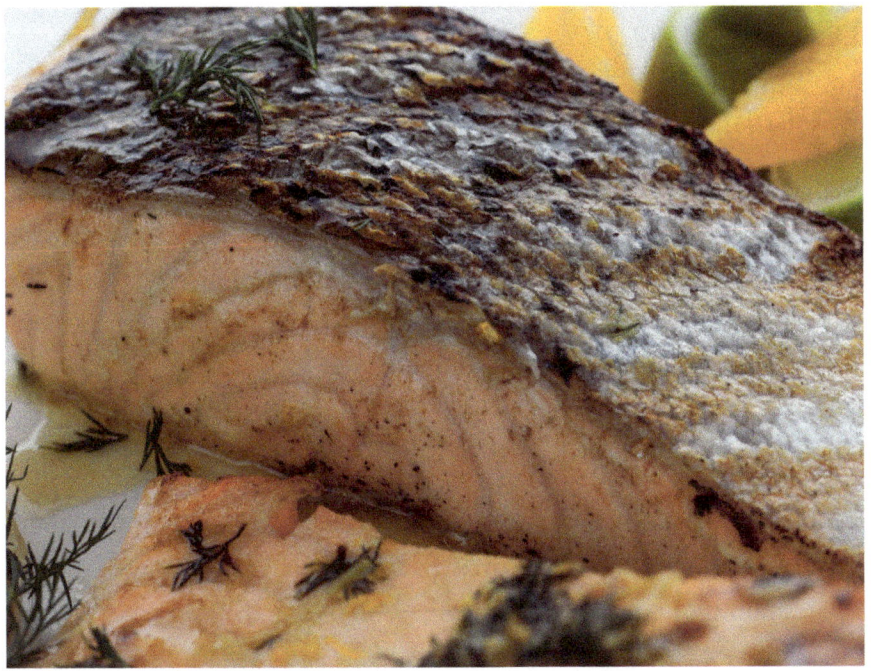

## Ingredients:

- $\frac{1}{4}$ cup brown sugar
- $\frac{1}{4}$ cup olive oil
- $\frac{1}{4}$ cup soy sauce
- 2 teaspoons lemon pepper

- 1 teaspoon dried thyme

- 1 teaspoon dried basil

- 1 teaspoon dried parsley

- $\frac{1}{2}$ teaspoon garlic powder

- 4 (6 ounce) salmon fillets

## Directions:

### Step 1

Whisk together the brown sugar, olive oil, soy sauce, lemon pepper, thyme, basil, parsley, and garlic powder in a bowl, and pour into a resealable plastic bag. Add the salmon fillets, coat with the marinade, squeeze out excess air, and seal the bag. Marinate in the refrigerator for at least 1 hour, turning occasionally.

### Step 2

Preheat an outdoor grill for medium heat, and lightly oil the grate. Remove the salmon from the marinade, and shake off excess. Discard the remaining marinade.

### Step 3

Grill the salmon on the preheated grill until browned and the fish flakes easily with a fork, about 5 minutes on each side.

Per Serving: 380 calories; protein 34.7g; carbohydrates 15.7g; fat 19.4g; cholesterol 87.8mg; sodium 1250.5mg.

# 21 - Grilled Salmon Honey-Ginger

| Preparation | Cooking | Servings |
|:---:|:---:|:---:|
| 10 min | 15 min | 4 |

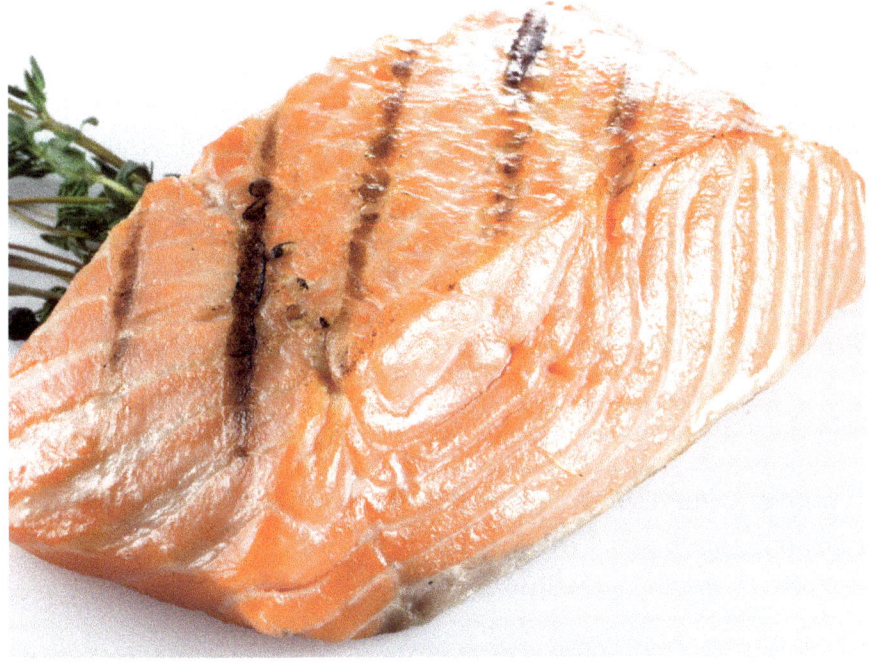

## Ingredients:

- 1 teaspoon ground ginger
- 1 teaspoon garlic powder
- ⅓ cup soy sauce
- ⅓ cup orange juice

- $\frac{1}{4}$ cup honey

- 1 green onion, chopped

- 1 (1 1/2-pound) salmon fillet

## Directions:

### Step 1

In a large self-closing plastic bag, combine ginger, garlic, soy sauce, orange juice, honey, and green onion; mix well. Place salmon in bag and seal tightly. Turn bag gently to distribute marinade. Refrigerate for 15 to 30 minutes.

### Step 2

Preheat an outdoor grill for medium heat and lightly oil grate.

### Step 3

Remove salmon from marinade, shake off excess, and discard remaining marinade. Grill for 12 to 15 minutes per inch of thickness, or until the fish flakes easily with a fork.

Per Serving: 373 calories; protein 37.6g; carbohydrates 22.3g; fat 14.5g; cholesterol 114mg; sodium 1291mg.

# 22 - Grilled Halibut with Cilantro
## Garlic Butter

| Preparation | Cooking | Servings |
|:---:|:---:|:---:|
| 25 min | 8 min | 4 |

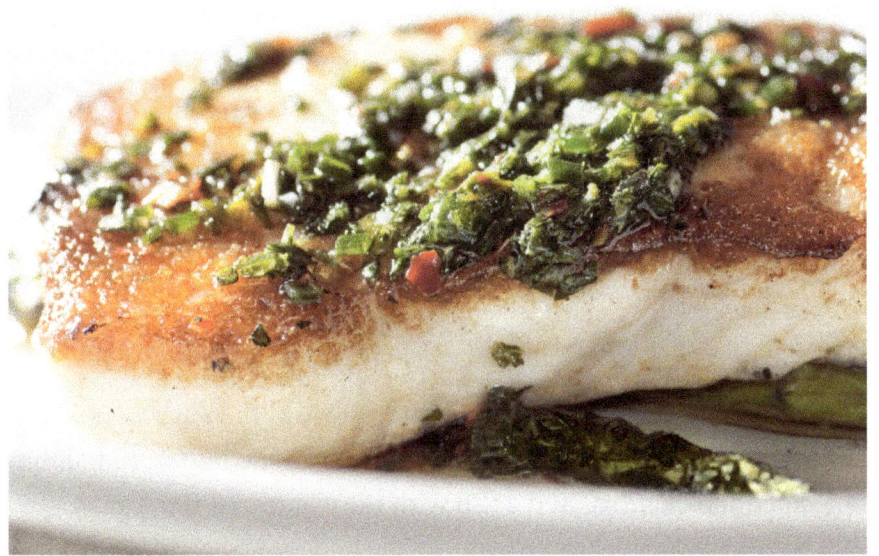

## Ingredients:

- 4 (6 ounce) fillets halibut
- 1 lime, cut into wedges
- salt and pepper to taste
- 3 cloves garlic, coarsely chopped

- $\frac{1}{2}$ cup chopped fresh cilantro

- 1 tablespoon fresh lime juice

- 2 tablespoons butter

- 1 tablespoon olive oil

## Directions:

### Step 1

Preheat a grill for high heat. Squeeze the juice from the lime wedges over fish fillets, then season them with salt and pepper.

### Step 2

Grill fish fillets for about 5 minutes on each side, until browned and fish can be flaked with a fork. Remove to a warm serving plate.

### Step 3

Heat the oil in a skillet over medium heat. Add the garlic; cook and stir just until fragrant, about 2 minutes. Stir in the butter, remaining lime juice and cilantro. Serve fish with the cilantro butter sauce.

Per Serving: 276 calories; protein 35.4g; carbohydrates 3g; fat 13.1g; cholesterol 69mg; sodium 173.9mg.

# 23 - Steaks Halibut Barbeque

| Preparation | Cooking | Servings |
|:---:|:---:|:---:|
| 10 min | 15 min | 4 |

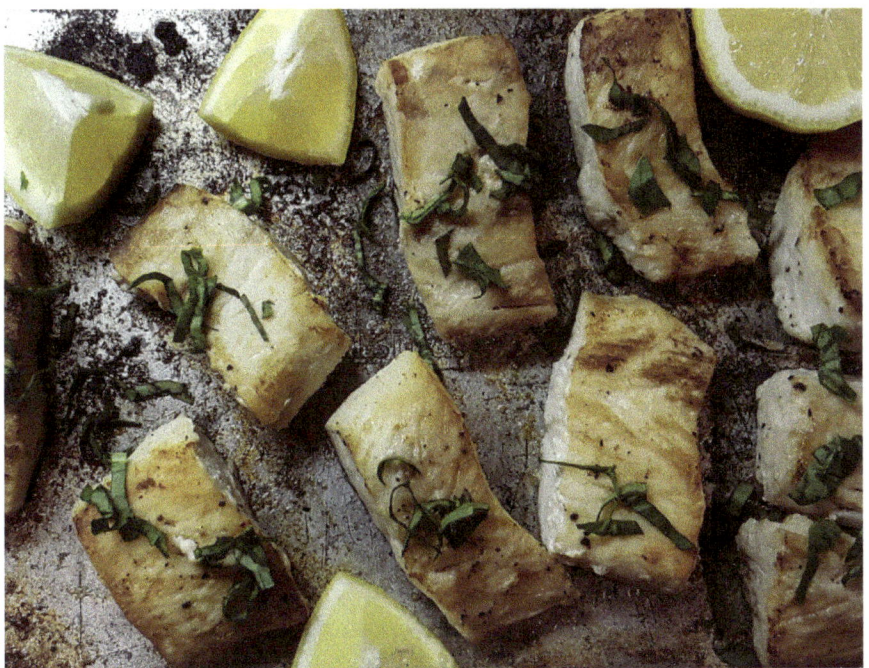

## Ingredients:

- 2 tablespoons butter
- 2 tablespoons brown sugar
- 2 cloves garlic, minced
- 1 tablespoon lemon juice

- 2 teaspoons soy sauce
- $\frac{1}{2}$ teaspoon ground black pepper
- 1 (1 pound) halibut steak

## Directions:

### Step 1

Preheat grill for medium-high heat.

### Step 2

Place butter, brown sugar, garlic, lemon juice, soy sauce, and pepper in a small saucepan. Warm over medium heat, stirring occasionally, until sugar is completely dissolved.

### Step 3

Lightly oil grill grate. Brush fish with brown sugar sauce, and place on grill. Cook for 5 minutes per side, or until fish can be easily flaked with a fork, basting with sauce. Discard remaining basting sauce.

Per Serving: 275 calories; protein 32g; carbohydrates 10.5g; fat 11.2g; cholesterol 68.8mg; sodium 338.3mg.

# 24 – Lemon Grilled Salmon

| Preparation | Cooking | Servings |
|:---:|:---:|:---:|
| 15 min | 15 min | 6 |

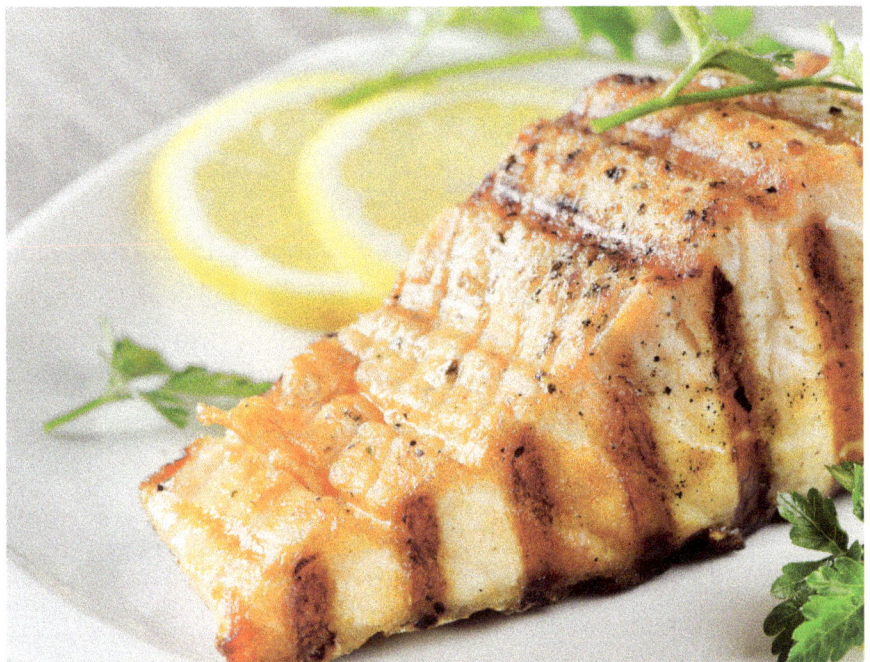

## Ingredients:

- $\frac{1}{2}$ cup olive oil
- $\frac{1}{4}$ cup lemon juice
- 4 green onions, thinly sliced
- 1 tablespoon chopped fresh parsley

- 1 teaspoon chopped fresh rosemary
- 1 teaspoon chopped fresh thyme
- $\frac{1}{2}$ teaspoon salt
- ⅛ teaspoon black pepper
- ⅛ teaspoon garlic powder
- 3 pounds salmon fillets

## Directions:

### Step 1

Combine olive oil, lemon juice, green onions, parsley, rosemary, thyme, salt, black pepper, and garlic powder in a small bowl. Set aside 1/4 cup of the marinade. Place salmon in a shallow dish and pour the remaining marinade over the top. Cover and refrigerate for 30 minutes. Remove the salmon and discard the used marinade.

### Step 2

Preheat grill for medium heat and lightly oil the grate.

### Step 3

Place salmon on the preheated grill skin side down. Cook, basting occasionally with the reserved marinade, until the fish flakes easily with a fork, 15 to 20 minutes.

Per Serving: 412 calories; protein 41.8g; carbohydrates 1.8g; fat 25.7g; cholesterol 97.4mg; sodium 299mg.

# 25 - Grilled Teriyaki Shrimp and
## Pineapple Skewers

| Preparation | Cooking | Servings |
| --- | --- | --- |
| 25 min | 20 min | 4 |

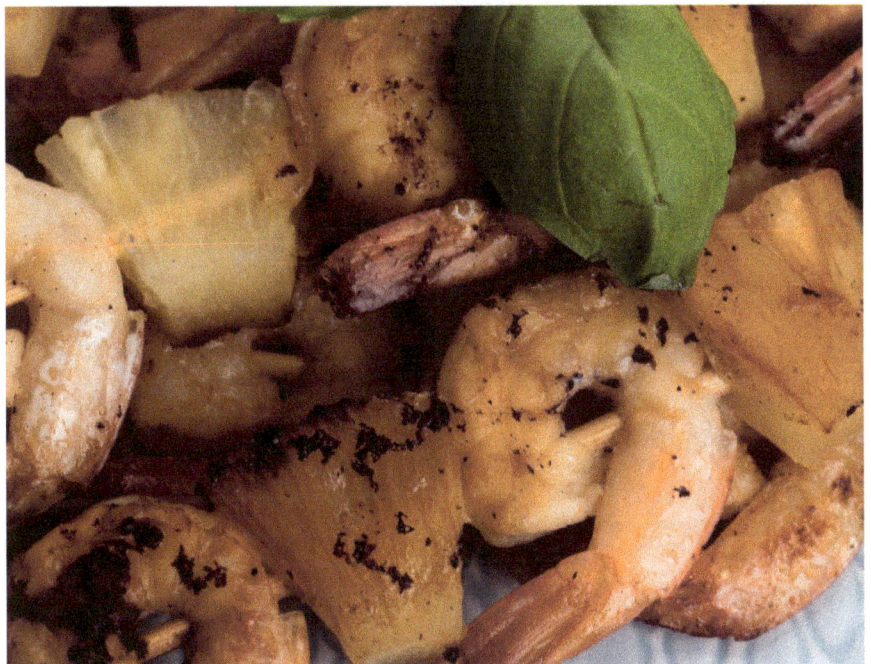

## Ingredients:

- ⅓ cup water
- 2 tablespoons soy sauce
- 2 tablespoons brown sugar
- 1 teaspoon honey

- 1 teaspoon grated fresh garlic

- 1 teaspoon grated fresh ginger

- 1 pound jumbo shrimp

- $\frac{1}{2}$ fresh pineapple, cored and cut into 1 1/2-inch pieces

- skewers

- 2 tablespoons minced fresh cilantro

- 1 tablespoon toasted sesame seeds

## Directions:

### Step 1

Combine water, soy sauce, brown sugar, honey, garlic, and ginger in a small saucepan and bring to a boil over medium-high heat. Reduce heat to medium-low and simmer until sauce has reduced and thickened slightly, 8 to 10 minutes.

### Step 2

Preheat an outdoor grill for medium-high heat and lightly oil grate. Thread shrimp and pineapple alternately onto skewers and place on a platter.

### Step 3

Arrange skewers on the hot grate. Grill 2 to 3 minutes per side, or until shrimp is opaque and cooked through. Turn grill to low heat and brush sauce on both sides of skewers. Transfer to a serving platter and sprinkle with cilantro and sesame seeds.

Per Serving: 223 calories; protein 20.4g; carbohydrates 32g; fat 2.3g; cholesterol 172.6mg; sodium 654.1mg.

# 26 - Halibut Fish Tacos

| Preparation | Cooking | Servings |
| --- | --- | --- |
| 20 min | 10 min | 8 |

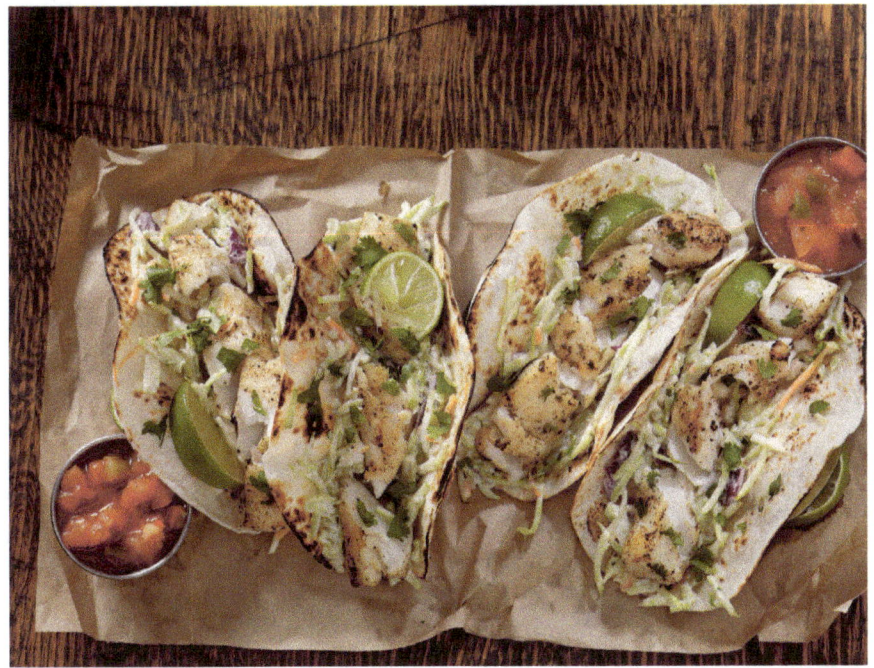

## Ingredients:

- 1 lime, juiced
- $\frac{1}{4}$ cup olive oil
- $\frac{1}{4}$ cup chopped cilantro
- 1 jalapeno pepper, diced

- 1 tablespoon ground ancho chile powder

- $\frac{1}{4}$ teaspoon ground cumin

- salt and ground black pepper to taste

- $\frac{1}{2}$ pound halibut fillets

- 8 corn tortillas

- Toppings:

- 2 cups shredded cabbage

- 1 (8 ounce) jar salsa

- 1 cup shredded pepper Jack cheese

- 1 avocado, sliced

## Directions:

### Step 1

Stir lime juice, olive oil, cilantro, jalapeno, chile powder, cumin, salt, and pepper together in a large bowl or resealable zip-top bag. Add halibut and marinate for 20 to 25 minutes. Do not over-marinate, as lime juice will start to 'cook' the fish.

### Step 2

Preheat an outdoor grill for medium heat and lightly oil the grate. Drain marinade; grill fillets for 5 minutes. Turn and cook until fish flakes easily with a fork, about 2 minutes more.

### Step 3

Warm tortillas on the grill or stove. Divide halibut among tortillas and top with cabbage, salsa, pepper Jack cheese, and avocado.

Per Serving: 269 calories; protein 12.4g; carbohydrates 18.2g; fat 17.1g; cholesterol 28.2mg; sodium 321.1mg.

# 27 - Spicy Grilled Shrimp

| Preparation | Cooking | Servings |
|:---:|:---:|:---:|
| 15 min | 7 min | 6 |

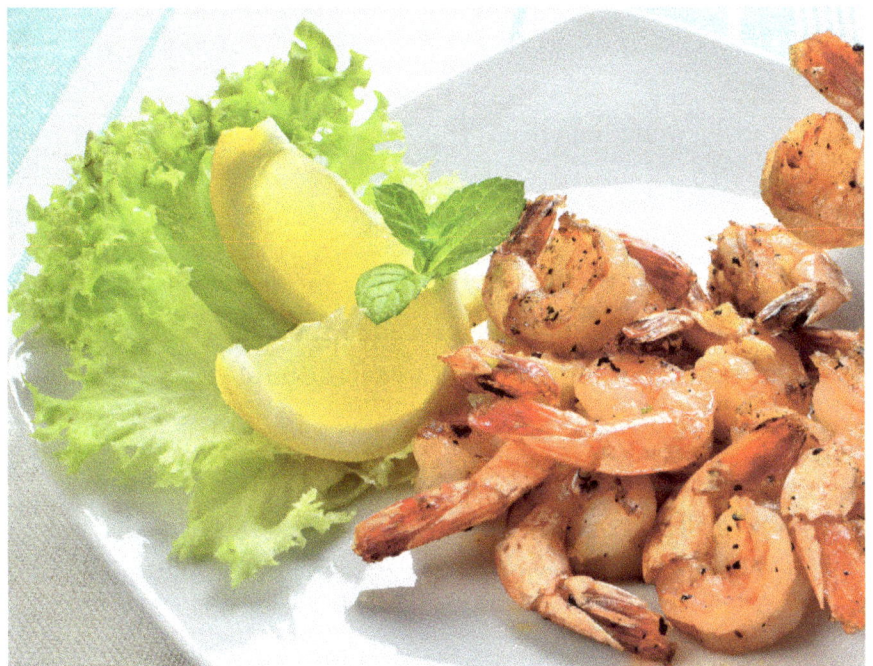

## Ingredients:

- 1 large clove garlic
- 1 teaspoon coarse salt
- $\frac{1}{2}$ teaspoon cayenne pepper
- 1 teaspoon paprika

- 2 tablespoons olive oil
- 2 teaspoons lemon juice
- 2 pounds large shrimp, peeled and deveined
- 8 wedges lemon, for garnish

## Directions:

### Step 1

Preheat grill for medium heat.

### Step 2

In a small bowl, crush the garlic with the salt. Mix in cayenne pepper and paprika, and then stir in olive oil and lemon juice to form a paste. In a large bowl, toss shrimp with garlic paste until evenly coated.

### Step 3

Lightly oil grill grate. Cook shrimp for 2 to 3 minutes per side, or until opaque. Transfer to a serving dish, garnish with lemon wedges, and serve.

Per Serving: 164 calories; protein 25.1g; carbohydrates 2.7g; fat 5.9g; cholesterol 230.4mg; sodium 585.7mg.

# 28 - Tuna Steak Marinated

| Preparation | Cooking | Servings |
|:---:|:---:|:---:|
| 10 min | 20 min | 4 |

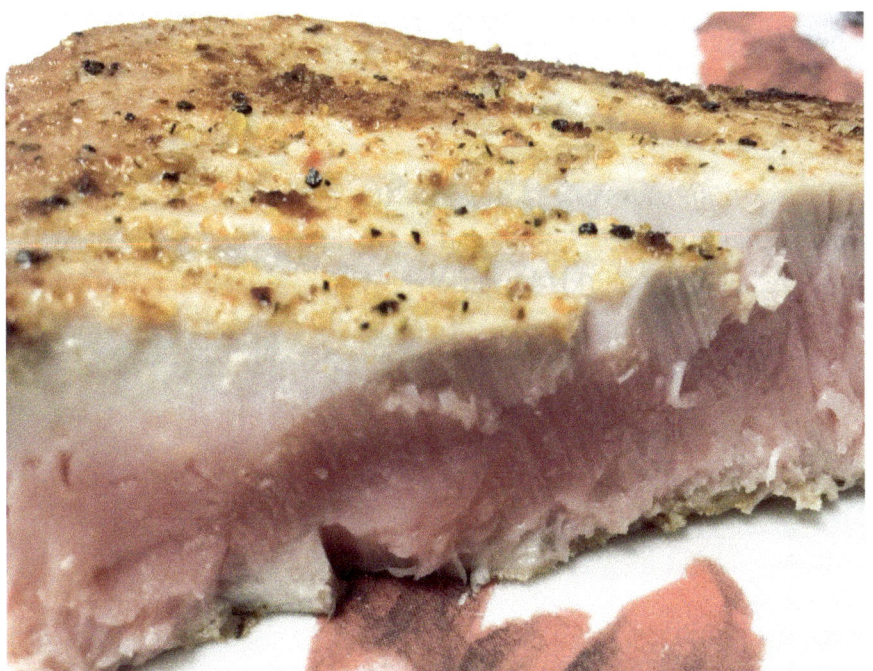

## Ingredients:

- $\frac{1}{4}$ cup orange juice
- $\frac{1}{4}$ cup soy sauce
- 2 tablespoons olive oil
- 1 tablespoon lemon juice

- 2 tablespoons chopped fresh parsley

- 1 clove garlic, minced

- $\frac{1}{2}$ teaspoon chopped fresh oregano

- $\frac{1}{2}$ teaspoon ground black pepper

- 4 (4 ounce) tuna steaks

## Directions:

## Step 1

In a large non-reactive dish, mix together the orange juice, soy sauce, olive oil, lemon juice, parsley, garlic, oregano, and pepper. Place the tuna steaks in the marinade and turn to coat. Cover, and refrigerate for at least 30 minutes.

## Step 2

Preheat grill for high heat.

## Step 3

Lightly oil grill grate. Cook the tuna steaks for 5 to 6 minutes, then turn and baste with the marinade. Cook for an additional 5 minutes, or to desired doneness. Discard any remaining marinade.

Per Serving: 200 calories; protein 27.4g; carbohydrates 3.7g; fat 7.9g; cholesterol 50.6mg; sodium 944.6mg.

# 29 - Grilled Salmon

| Preparation | Cooking | Servings |
| --- | --- | --- |
| 15 min | 16 min | 6 |

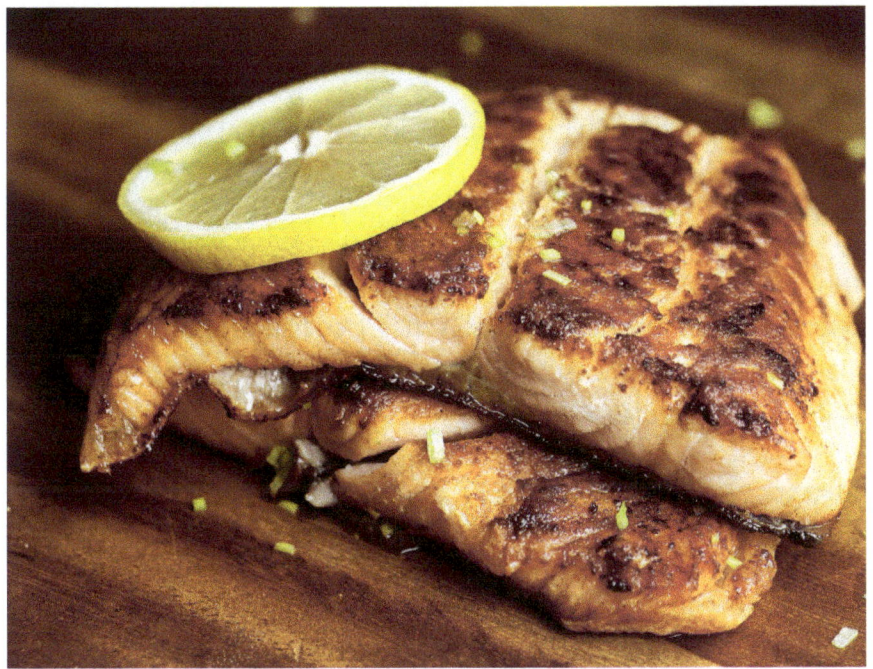

## Ingredients:

- 1 $\frac{1}{2}$ pounds salmon fillets
- lemon pepper to taste
- garlic powder to taste
- salt to taste

- ⅓ cup soy sauce
- ⅓ cup brown sugar
- ⅓ cup water
- ¼ cup vegetable oil

## Directions:

### Step 1

Season salmon fillets with lemon pepper, garlic powder, and salt.

### Step 2

In a small bowl, stir together soy sauce, brown sugar, water, and vegetable oil until sugar is dissolved. Place fish in a large resealable plastic bag with the soy sauce mixture, seal, and turn to coat. Refrigerate for at least 2 hours.

### Step 3

Preheat grill for medium heat.

### Step 4

Lightly oil grill grate. Place salmon on the preheated grill, and discard marinade. Cook salmon for 6 to 8 minutes per side, or until the fish flakes easily with a fork.

Per Serving: 318 calories; protein 20.5g; carbohydrates 13.2g; fat 20.1g; cholesterol 55.8mg; sodium 1091.8mg.

# 30 - Salmon Cedar Planked

| Preparation | Cooking | Servings |
|:---:|:---:|:---:|
| 15 min | 20 min | 6 |

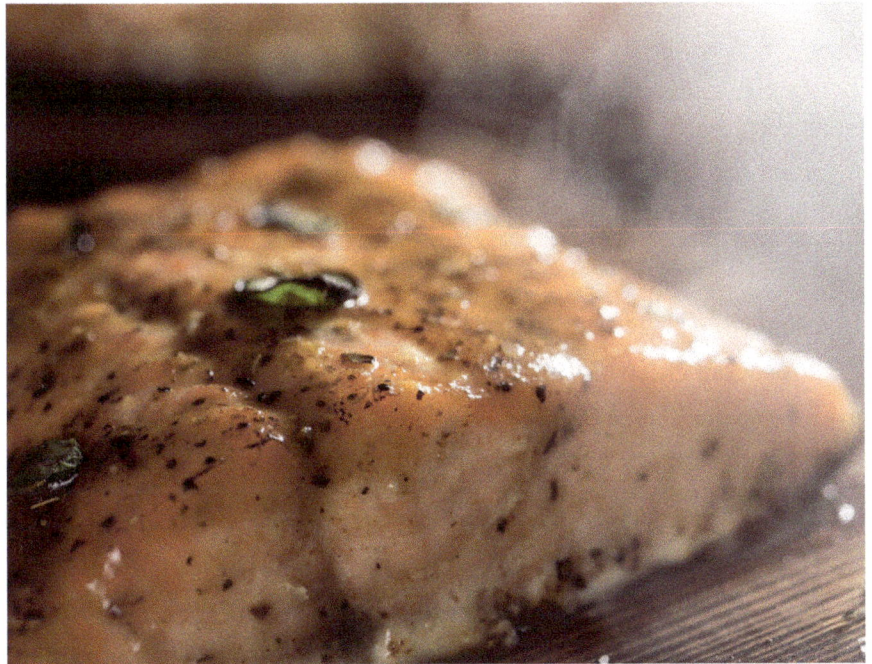

## Ingredients:

- 3 (12 inch) untreated cedar planks
- ⅓ cup vegetable oil
- 1 ½ tablespoons rice vinegar
- 1 teaspoon sesame oil
- ⅓ cup soy sauce

- $\frac{1}{4}$ cup chopped green onions
- 1 tablespoon grated fresh ginger root
- 1 teaspoon minced garlic
- 2 (2 pound) salmon fillets, skin removed

## Directions:

### Step 1

Soak the cedar planks for at least 1 hour in warm water. Soak longer if you have time.

### Step 2

In a shallow dish, stir together the vegetable oil, rice vinegar, sesame oil, soy sauce, green onions, ginger, and garlic. Place the salmon fillets in the marinade and turn to coat. Cover and marinate for at least 15 minutes, or up to one hour.

### Step 3

Preheat an outdoor grill for medium heat. Place the planks on the grate. The boards are ready when they start to smoke and crackle just a little.

### Step 4

Place the salmon fillets onto the planks and discard the marinade. Cover, and grill for about 20 minutes. Fish is done when you can flake it with a fork. It will continue to cook after you remove it from the grill.

Per Serving: 678 calories; protein 61.3g; carbohydrates 1.7g; fat 45.8g; cholesterol 178.6mg; sodium 981.2mg.

# 31 - Marinated Grilled Shrimp

| Preparation | Cooking | Servings |
|:---:|:---:|:---:|
| 30 min | 10 min | 6 |

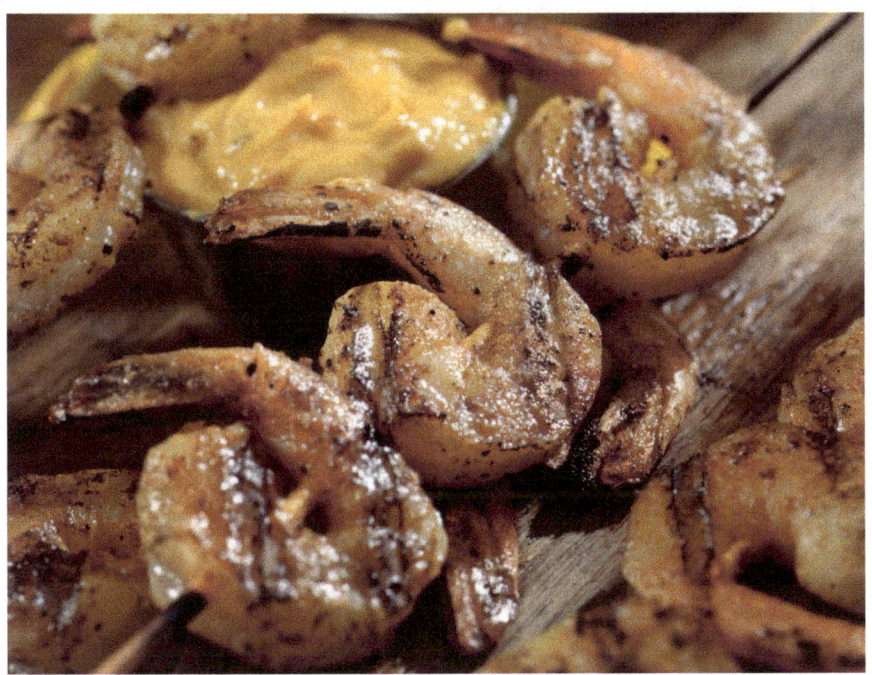

## Ingredient:

- 1 cup olive oil
- $\frac{1}{4}$ cup chopped fresh parsley
- 1 lemon, juiced
- 2 tablespoons hot pepper sauce

- 3 cloves garlic, minced
- 1 tablespoon tomato paste
- 2 teaspoons dried oregano
- 1 teaspoon salt
- 1 teaspoon ground black pepper
- 2 pounds large shrimp, peeled and deveined with tails attached
- 6 each skewers

## Directions:

### Step 1

In a mixing bowl, mix together olive oil, parsley, lemon juice, hot sauce, garlic, tomato paste, oregano, salt, and black pepper. Reserve a small amount for basting later. Pour remaining marinade into a large resealable plastic bag with shrimp. Seal, and marinate in the refrigerator for 2 hours.

### Step 2

Preheat grill for medium-low heat. Thread shrimp onto skewers, piercing once near the tail and once near the head. Discard marinade.

### Step 3

Lightly oil grill grate. Cook shrimp for 5 minutes per side, or until opaque, basting frequently with reserved marinade.

Per Serving: 447 calories; protein 25.3g; carbohydrates 3.7g; fat 37.5g; cholesterol 230.4mg; sodium 800mg.

# 32 - Yellow Tuna Grilled Marinade

| Preparation | Cooking | Servings |
|:---:|:---:|:---:|
| 10 min | 14 min | 4 |

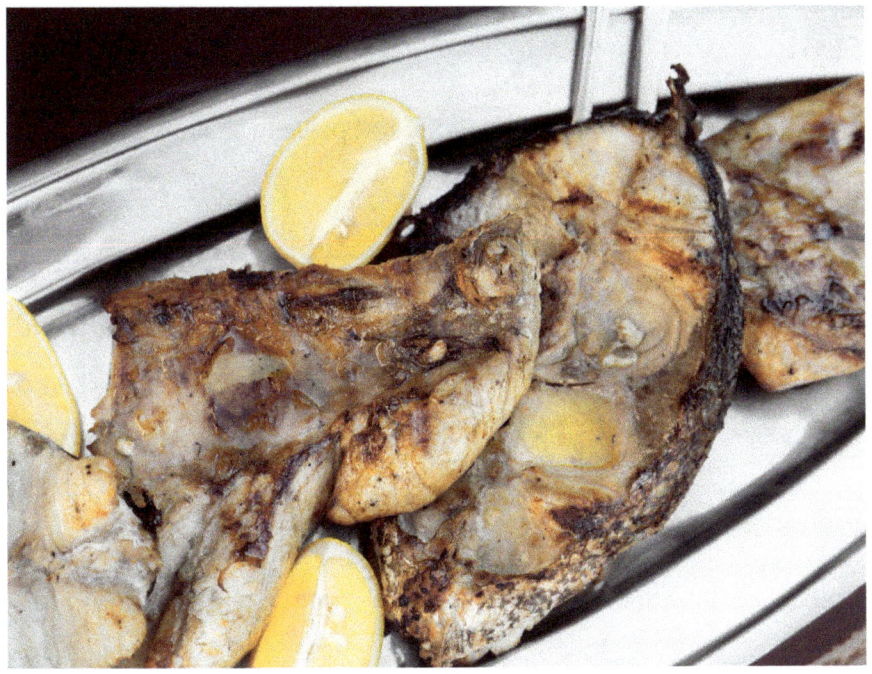

## Ingredients:

- 4 (6 ounce) yellowfin tuna steaks
- ½ cup vegetable oil
- ⅓ cup soy sauce
- ¼ cup fresh lemon juice

- 2 teaspoons Dijon mustard
- 1 teaspoon grated lemon peel
- 1 clove garlic, crushed
- 4 wedges lemon, for garnish

## Directions:

### Step 1

Prick tuna steaks all over with a fork and place in shallow glass dish.

### Step 2

Whisk oil, soy sauce, lemon juice, Dijon mustard, lemon peel, and garlic together in a bowl; pour over the tuna steaks. Cover dish with plastic wrap and refrigerate 1 to 3 hours.

### Step 3

Preheat grill for medium heat and lightly oil the grate.

### Step 4

Remove tuna from the marinade. Shake excess moisture from the steaks.

### Step 5

Pour the marinade into a small saucepan and bring to a boil. Reduce heat to medium-low and cook marinade at a simmer for 10 minutes.

## Step 6

Cook tuna on preheated grill, basting with boiled marinade, until cooked through, 5 to 6 minutes per side. Serve with lemon wedges.

Per Serving: 448 calories; protein 41.5g; carbohydrates 5.2g; fat 28.9g; cholesterol 77.1mg; sodium 1328.3mg.

# 33 - Cajun Blackened Catfish

| Preparation | Cooking | Servings |
|:---:|:---:|:---:|
| 10 min | 12 min | 4 |

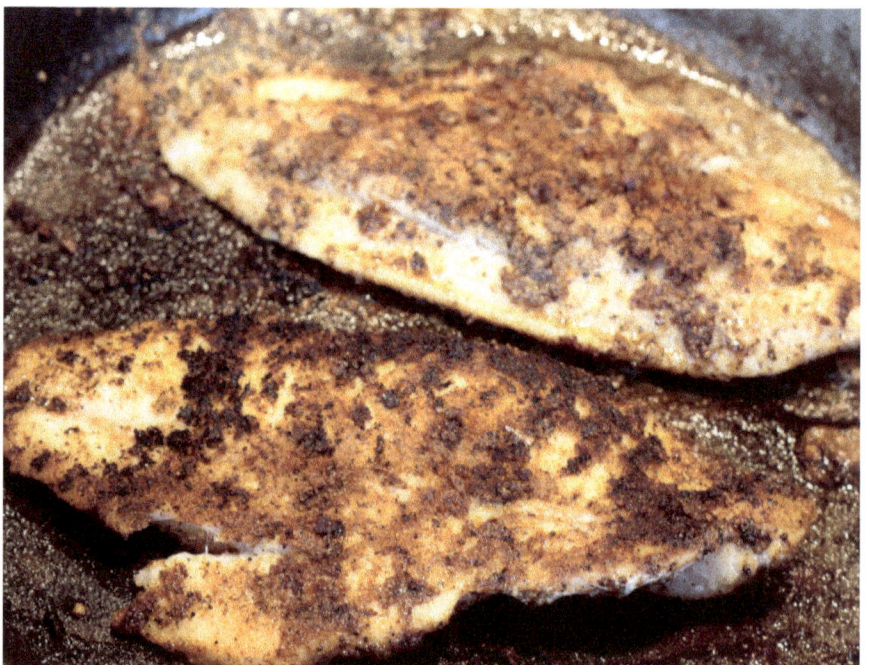

## Ingredients:

- 1 teaspoon ground black pepper
- 1 teaspoon garlic powder
- 1 teaspoon onion powder
- 1 teaspoon paprika

- 1 teaspoon dried parsley
- 1 teaspoon ground cayenne pepper
- 1 teaspoon kosher salt
- $\frac{1}{2}$ teaspoon dried oregano
- $\frac{1}{2}$ teaspoon dried thyme
- 4 (4 ounce) catfish fillets, skinned
- $\frac{3}{4}$ cup unsalted butter

## Directions:

### Step 1

In a shallow bowl, mix together the black pepper, garlic powder, onion powder, paprika, parsley, cayenne pepper, kosher salt, oregano, and thyme until thoroughly combined. Press the catfish fillets into the spice mixture to thoroughly coat.

### Step 2

Arrange a portable heat source outdoors, such as a butane burner or side burner of a gas grill. Melt butter in a glass or metal bowl. Light the burner, and place a large cast-iron skillet onto the burner over high heat. Pour about 1/4 cup of melted butter into the skillet; set remaining 1/2 cup of butter aside.

### Step 3

When the butter in the skillet is smoking hot, lay the catfish fillets into the skillet. Cook until the spices are burned onto the fillets and the catfish is opaque and flaky inside, about 3 minutes per side. Don't breathe smoke from burning spices. To serve, pour remaining 1/2 cup of butter over the catfish.

Per Serving: 466 calories; protein 18.2g; carbohydrates 2.2g; fat 43.2g; cholesterol 144.1mg; sodium 545.7mg.

# 34 - Grilled Octopus

| Preparation | Cooking | Servings |
|:---:|:---:|:---:|
| 15 min | 55 min | 6 |

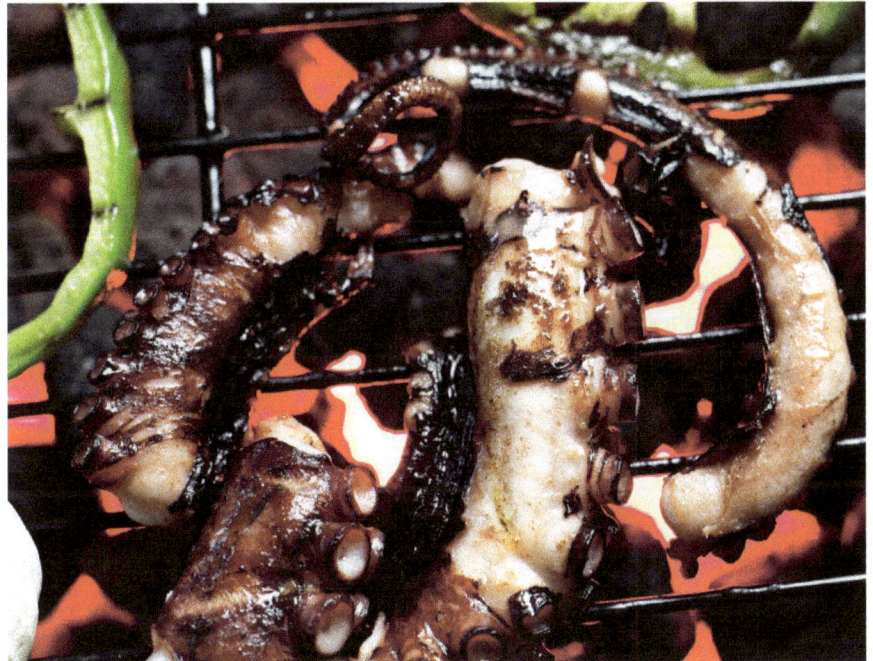

## Ingredients:

- 2 tablespoons kosher salt

- 1 tablespoon black peppercorns

- 1 wine cork

- 3 $\frac{1}{2}$ pounds octopus, head and beak removed

- 2 tablespoons extra virgin olive oil

- $\frac{1}{2}$ lemon

- $\frac{1}{2}$ tablespoon minced fresh parsley

- 1 pinch salt and freshly ground black pepper to taste

## Directions:

### Step 1

Fill a large pot 1/2 full with water. Add 2 tablespoons kosher salt, peppercorns, and the wine cork; bring to a boil over high heat.

### Step 2

Meanwhile, place octopus on a cutting board. Using a wooden spoon or meat mallet, pound the octopus multiple times, starting in the middle and moving down each tentacle to tenderize the meat.

### Step 3

Dip tentacles into the boiling water 3 times, holding them in the boiling water 2 to 3 seconds each time, until the tentacles curl up. Submerge entire octopus in the boiling water. Bring water back to a boil, reduce heat to low, cover, and simmer until octopus is fork-tender, 45 to 60 minutes. Remove from heat and cool for 30 minutes.

### Step 4

Preheat an outdoor grill for medium-high heat and lightly oil the grate.

## Step 5

Grill octopus until charred on all sides, 3 to 4 minutes per side.

## Step 6

Remove from heat, slice into pieces, and place on a serving platter. Drizzle with extra virgin olive oil, squeeze lemon over top, sprinkle with parsley, and season with salt and pepper to taste. Serve immediately.

**Per Serving: 384 calories; protein 61.9g; carbohydrates 10.6g; fat 8.9g; cholesterol 198.7mg; sodium 2898.9mg.**

# 35 - Grilled Rock Lobster Tails

| Preparation | Cooking | Servings |
|:---:|:---:|:---:|
| 15 min | 15 min | 4 |

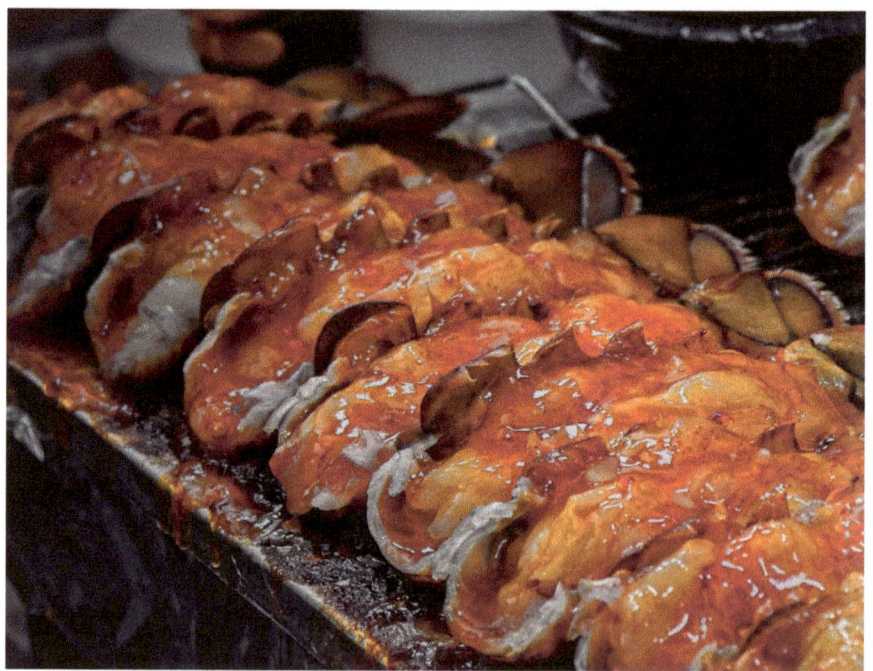

## Ingredients:

- 1 tablespoon lemon juice
- $\frac{1}{2}$ cup olive oil
- 1 teaspoon salt
- 1 teaspoon paprika

- ⅛ teaspoon white pepper
- ⅛ teaspoon garlic powder
- 4 (20 ounce) rock lobster tails

## Directions:

### Step 1

Preheat grill for high heat.

### Step 2

Squeeze lemon juice into a small bowl, and slowly whisk in olive oil. Whisk in salt, paprika, white pepper, and garlic powder. Split lobster tails lengthwise with a large knife, and brush flesh side of tail with marinade.

### Step 3

Lightly oil grill grate. Place tails, flesh side down, on preheated grill. Cook for 10 to 15 minutes, turning once, and basting frequently with marinade. Discard any remaining marinade. Lobster is done when opaque and firm to the touch.

Per Serving: 742 calories; protein 44.3g; carbohydrates 4.3g; fat 60.9g; cholesterol 169.3mg; sodium 2036mg.

# 36 - Grilled Halibut

| Preparation | Cooking | Servings |
|:---:|:---:|:---:|
| 10 min | 10 min | 4 |

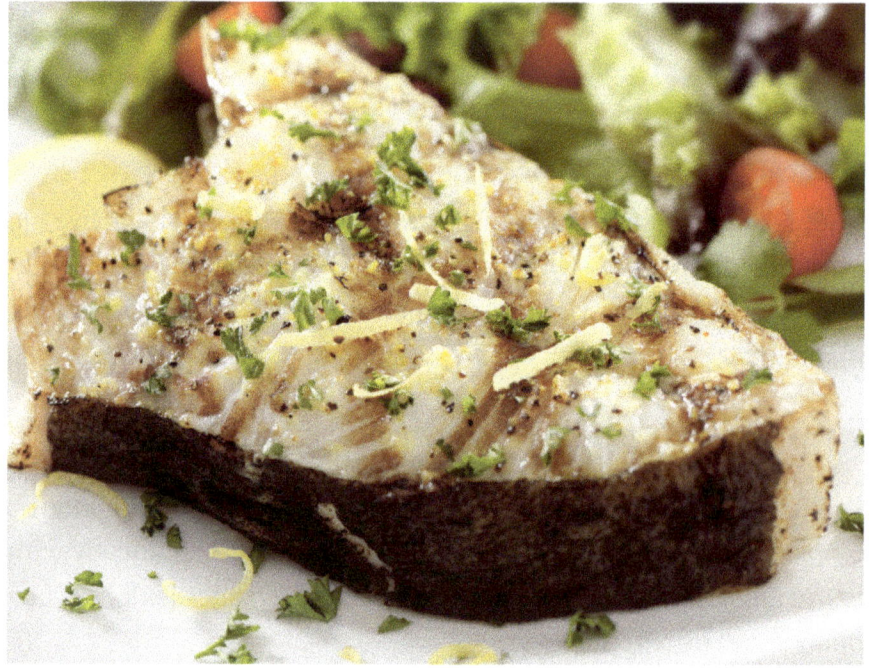

## Ingredients:

- $\frac{3}{4}$ cup butter, softened

- 1 tablespoon lemon juice

- 1 $\frac{1}{2}$ teaspoons onion powder

- 1 $\frac{1}{2}$ teaspoons dried parsley

- $\frac{3}{4}$ teaspoon dried dill weed (Optional)
- $\frac{1}{4}$ teaspoon white sugar (Optional)
- $\frac{1}{4}$ teaspoon salt
- $\frac{1}{4}$ teaspoon ground black pepper
- 4 inch-thick halibut steaks

## Directions:

Step 1

Preheat grill for medium heat and lightly oil the grate.

## Step 2

Stir butter, lemon juice, onion powder, parsley, dill, sugar, salt, and pepper together in a bowl; spread evenly over the halibut steaks.

## Step 3

Cook on preheated grill until the fish flakes easily with a fork, 5 to 6 minutes per side.

Per Serving: 498 calories; protein 36.4g; carbohydrates 1.5g; fat 37.7g; cholesterol 153.9mg; sodium 485.8mg.

# 37 - Swordfish Grilled Marinated

| Preparation | Cooking | Servings |
|:---:|:---:|:---:|
| 10 min | 15 min | 4 |

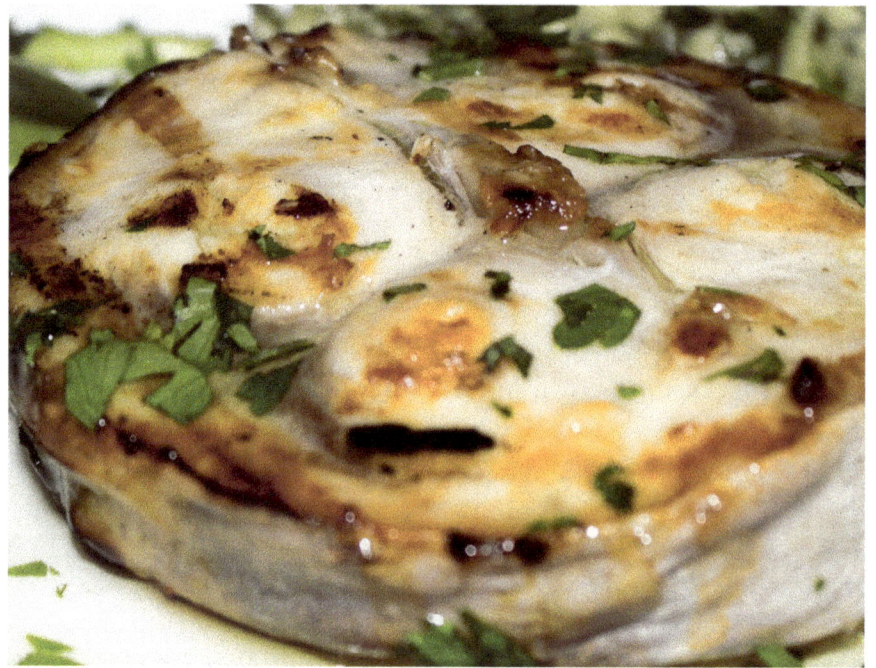

## Ingredients:

- 4 cloves garlic
- ⅓ cup white wine
- ¼ cup lemon juice
- 2 tablespoons soy sauce

- 2 tablespoons olive oil
- 1 tablespoon poultry seasoning
- $\frac{1}{4}$ teaspoon salt
- ⅛ teaspoon pepper
- 4 swordfish steaks
- 1 tablespoon chopped fresh parsley
- 4 slices lemon, for garnish

## Directions:

### Step 1

In a glass baking dish, combine the garlic, white wine, lemon juice, soy sauce, olive oil, poultry seasoning, salt and pepper. Mix just to blend. Place swordfish steaks into the marinade, and refrigerate for 1 hour, turning frequently.

### Step 2

Preheat an outdoor grill for high heat, and lightly oil the grate.

### Step 3

Grill swordfish steaks for 5 to 6 minutes on each side. Garnish with parsley and lemon wedges.

Per Serving: 258 calories; protein 27.6g; carbohydrates 5.6g; fat 12.3g; cholesterol 52.3mg; sodium 708mg.

# 38 - Grilled Garlic and Herb Shrimp

| Preparation | Cooking | Servings |
|:---:|:---:|:---:|
| 15 min | 8 min | 6 |

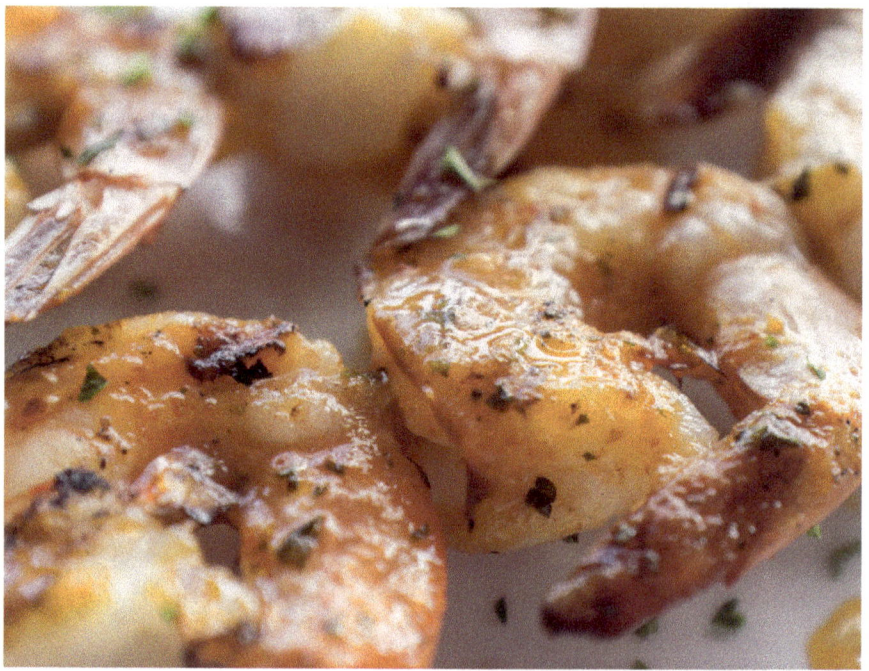

## Ingredients:

- 1 $\frac{1}{2}$ teaspoons kosher salt

- $\frac{1}{2}$ teaspoon lemon zest

- 3 cloves garlic, thinly sliced

- 3 tablespoons chopped fresh basil leaves

- 3 tablespoons chopped fresh flat-leaf parsley

- 1 tablespoon chopped fresh oregano leaves
- 1 tablespoon chopped fresh lemon thyme leaves
- 4 tablespoons olive oil, divided, or as needed
- 2 pounds extra large shrimp (16-20), peeled and deveined, tail left on
- skewers

## Sauce:

- 1 tablespoon olive oil
- $\frac{1}{2}$ lemon, juiced
- $\frac{1}{2}$ teaspoon red pepper flakes
- 1 pinch cayenne pepper
- salt and ground black pepper to taste
- 1 lemon, cut into wedges

## Directions:

### Step 1

Place salt, lemon zest, and 3 cloves garlic in bowl of a mortar and pestle. Pound with the pestle until mixture begins to form a paste, about 2 minutes. Add chopped basil, parsley, oregano, and thyme and pound with pestle until mixture begin to come together, about 5 minutes.

### Step 2

Drizzle about 1 tablespoon of the olive oil into herb mixture. Grind together until mixture begins to form a sauce for marinating, about 1 minute. Pour in the remaining 3 tablespoons olive oil. Stir mixture with a spoon until mixture is thoroughly combined, adding additional olive oil as needed. Mixture should be fairly thick but pourable.

## Step 3

Place shrimp in a large bowl and mix in about 2/3 of the sauce, reserving 1/3 for serving. Stir until shrimp are evenly coated with the sauce, about 2 minutes. Transfer shrimp to a resealable plastic bag. Refrigerate 2 to 3 hours. Cover and refrigerate remaining sauce.

## Step 4

Preheat an outdoor grill for high heat and lightly oil the grate.

## Step 5

Thread shrimp onto skewers (pierce each twice, once through large part of shrimp, once through small part). Place skewers on hot grill. Cook on each side until shrimp are bright pink and opaque and exterior is beginning to caramelize, 2 to 3 minutes per side. Transfer skewers to serving platter.

## Step 6

Pour remaining sauce into mixing bowl. Whisk in 1 tablespoon olive oil, lemon juice, red pepper flakes, cayenne pepper, salt and black pepper. Spoon sauce over shrimp. Serve with lemon wedges.

Per Serving: 223 calories; protein 25.1g; carbohydrates 1.9g; fat 12.6g; cholesterol 230.4mg; sodium 772.5mg.

# 39 - Maui Shrimp

| Preparation | Cooking | Servings |
|:---:|:---:|:---:|
| 15 min | 10 min | 6 |

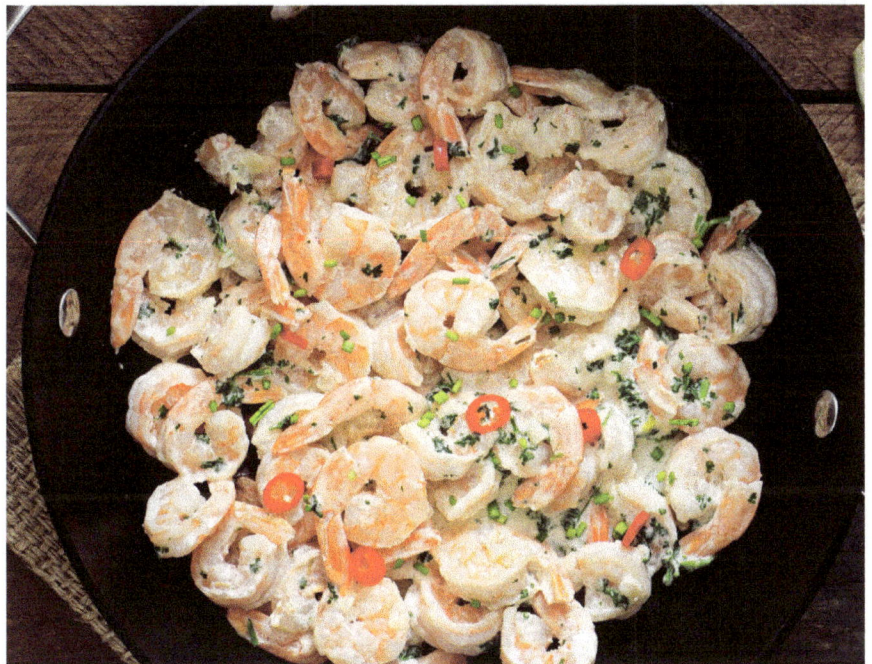

## Ingredients:

- 2 pounds uncooked medium shrimp, peeled and deveined
- 1 pinch garlic salt, or to taste
- ground black pepper to taste
- $\frac{1}{4}$ teaspoon cayenne pepper, or to taste (Optional)

- 1 cup mayonnaise
- 1 lemon, cut into wedges

## Directions:

### Step 1

Preheat outdoor grill for medium heat, and lightly oil the grate.

### Step 2

Thread shrimp onto skewers. Season both sides of shrimp with garlic salt and black pepper; if using cayenne, see Cook's Note.

### Step 3

Generously coat both sides of shrimp with mayonnaise.

### Step 4

Cook shrimp on heated grill until shrimp are bright pink on the outside and opaque on the inside, and the mayonnaise turns golden brown, 5 to 10 minutes on each side. Serve with lemon wedges.

Per Serving: 381 calories; protein 25.1g; carbohydrates 1.3g; fat 30.4g; cholesterol 244.4mg; sodium 528mg.

# 40 - Grilled Potato Salad

| Preparation | Cooking | Servings |
|:---:|:---:|:---:|
| 15 min | 40 min | 8 |

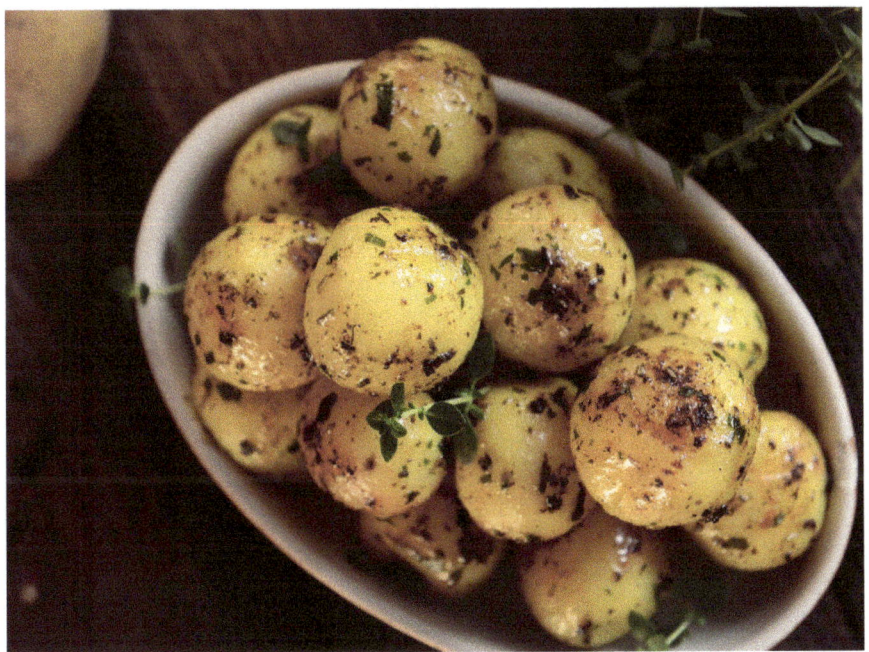

## Ingredients:

- 2 pounds red potatoes
- 2 tablespoons extra-virgin olive oil

  **Dressing**:
- ½ cup extra-virgin olive oil

- 1 tablespoon apple cider vinegar
- 1 teaspoon kosher salt
- 1 teaspoon ground black pepper
- 1 clove garlic, chopped
- $\frac{1}{2}$ teaspoon white sugar
- 6 slices cooked bacon, chopped
- 4 green onions, chopped
- 2 tablespoons minced fresh parsley

## Directions:

### Step 1

Preheat grill for medium heat and lightly oil the grate.

### Step 2

Place potatoes in a bowl; add 2 tablespoons olive oil and toss to coat.

### Step 3

Cook on preheated grill until tender, about 30 minutes. Cool potatoes, 10 to 15 minutes; cut into quarters.

### Step 4

Whisk 1/2 cup olive oil, vinegar, salt, black pepper, garlic, and sugar together in a bowl until dressing is smooth. Toss potatoes, bacon, green onions, and parsley with dressing in a bowl until evenly coated.

Per Serving: 290 calories; protein 5.7g; carbohydrates 19.4g; fat 21.3g; cholesterol 9.9mg; sodium 456.7mg

# 41 - Grilled Asparagus

| Preparation | Cooking | Servings |
|:---:|:---:|:---:|
| 15 min | 4 min | 4 |

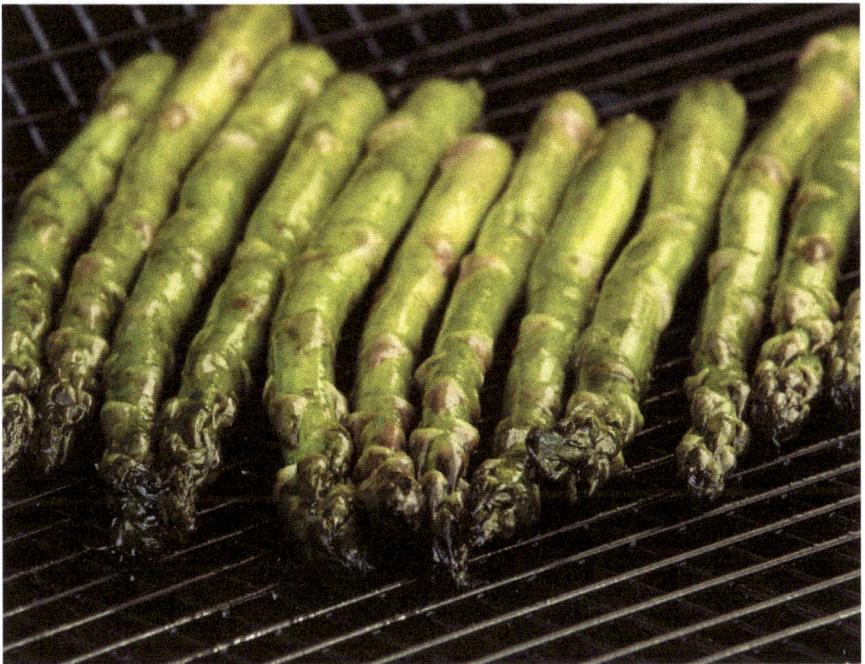

## Ingredients:

- 1 pound fresh asparagus spears, trimmed
- 1 tablespoon olive oil
- salt and pepper to taste

## Directions:

### Step 1

Preheat grill for high heat.

### Step 2

Lightly coat the asparagus spears with olive oil. Season with salt and pepper to taste.

### Step 3

Grill over high heat for 2 to 3 minutes, or to desired tenderness.

Per Serving: 53 calories; protein 2.5g; carbohydrates 4.4g; fat 3.5g; sodium 2.3mg.

# 42 – Brazilian Grilled Pineapple

| Preparation | Cooking | Servings |
| --- | --- | --- |
| 10 min | 10 min | 6 |

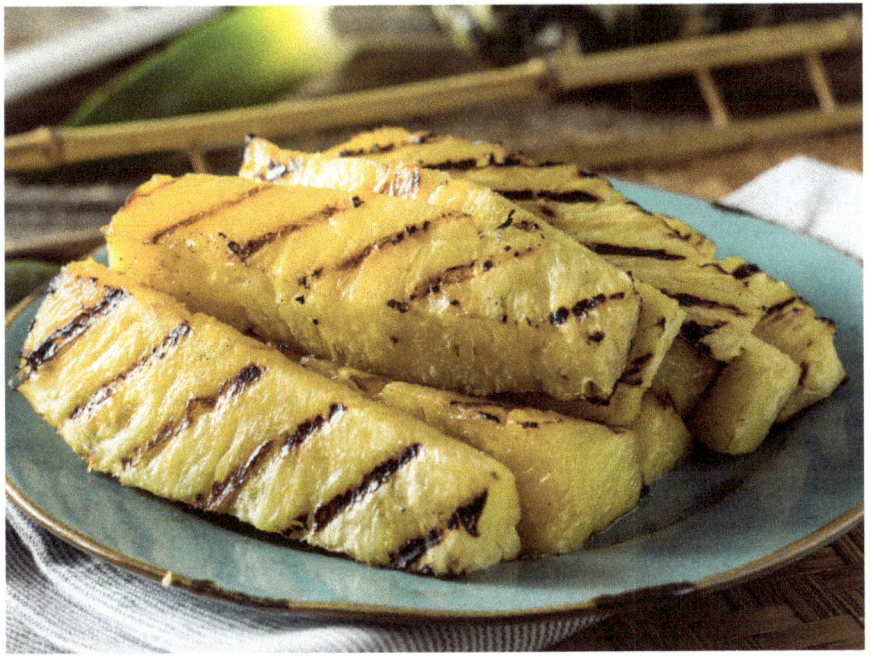

## Ingredients:

- 1 cup brown sugar
- 2 teaspoons ground cinnamon
- 1 pineapple - peeled, cored, and cut into 6 wedges

## Directions:

### Step 1

Preheat an outdoor grill for medium-high heat and lightly oil the grate.

### Step 2

Whisk brown sugar and cinnamon together in a bowl. Pour sugar mixture into a large resealable plastic bag. Place pineapple wedges in bag and shake to coat each wedge.

### Step 3

Grill pineapple wedges on the preheated grill until heated through, 3 to 5 minutes per side.

Per Serving: 255 calories; protein 1.3g; carbohydrates 66.4g; fat 0.3g; sodium 12.6mg.

# 43 – Honey Grilled Pineapple

| Preparation | Cooking | Servings |
|:-----------:|:-------:|:--------:|
| 5 min | 10 min | 8 |

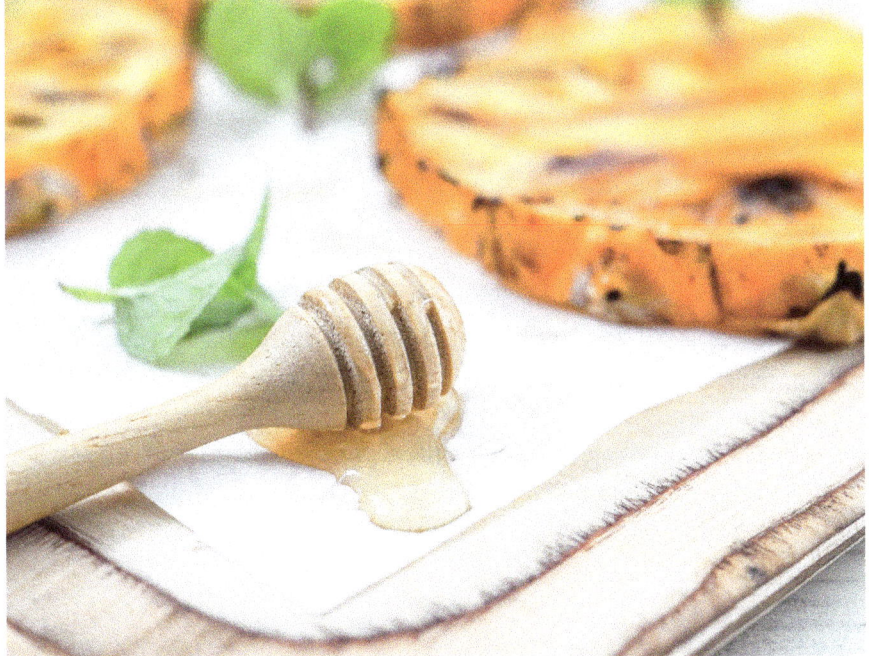

## Ingredients:

- 1 fresh pineapple - peeled, cored and cut into 1-inch rings
- 1 teaspoon honey
- 3 tablespoons melted butter
- 1 dash hot pepper sauce

- salt to taste

## Directions:

### Step 1

Place pineapple in a large resealable plastic bag. Add honey, butter, hot pepper sauce, and salt. Seal bag, and shake to coat evenly. Marinate for at least 30 minutes, or preferably overnight.

### Step 2

Preheat an outdoor grill for high heat, and lightly oil grate.

### Step 3

Grill pineapple for 2 to 3 minutes per side, or until heated through and grill marks appear.

Per Serving: 46 calories; protein 0.2g; carbohydrates 5.3g; fat 2.9g; cholesterol 7.6mg; sodium 23.1mg.

# 44 - Grilled Bell Peppers

| Preparation | Cooking | Servings |
|:-----------:|:-------:|:--------:|
| 15 min | 15 min | 6 |

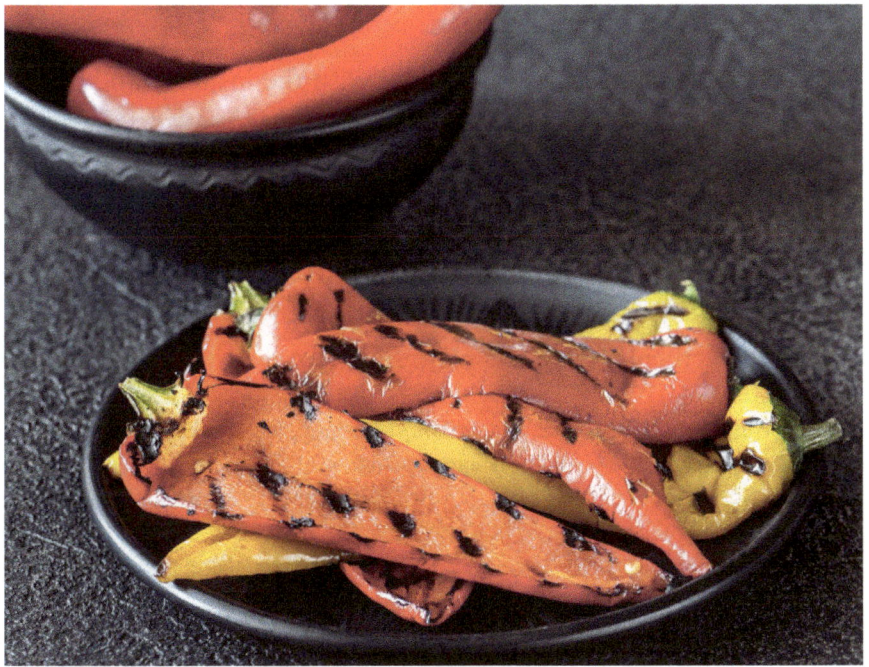

## Ingredients:

- 3 green bell peppers, cut into large chunks
- $\frac{1}{2}$ cup sliced jalapeno peppers
- 1 pinch dried oregano
- 1 cup shredded mozzarella cheese

## Directions:

### Step 1

Preheat a grill for medium-high heat. When the grill is hot, lightly oil the grate.

### Step 2

Place the pepper pieces onto the grill with the inside facing down. Cook until slightly charred, 3 to 5 minutes.

### Step 3

Turn peppers over, and place jalapeno slices onto them. Top with some mozzarella cheese, and sprinkle with a bit of oregano. Grill until cheese melts, then remove to a plate and serve.

Per Serving: 63 calories; protein 5.2g; carbohydrates 3.9g; fat 3.2g; cholesterol 12.1mg; sodium 307.8mg.

# 45 - Easy Roasted Cabbage

| Preparation | Cooking | Servings |
|:---:|:---:|:---:|
| 10 min | 40 min | 6 |

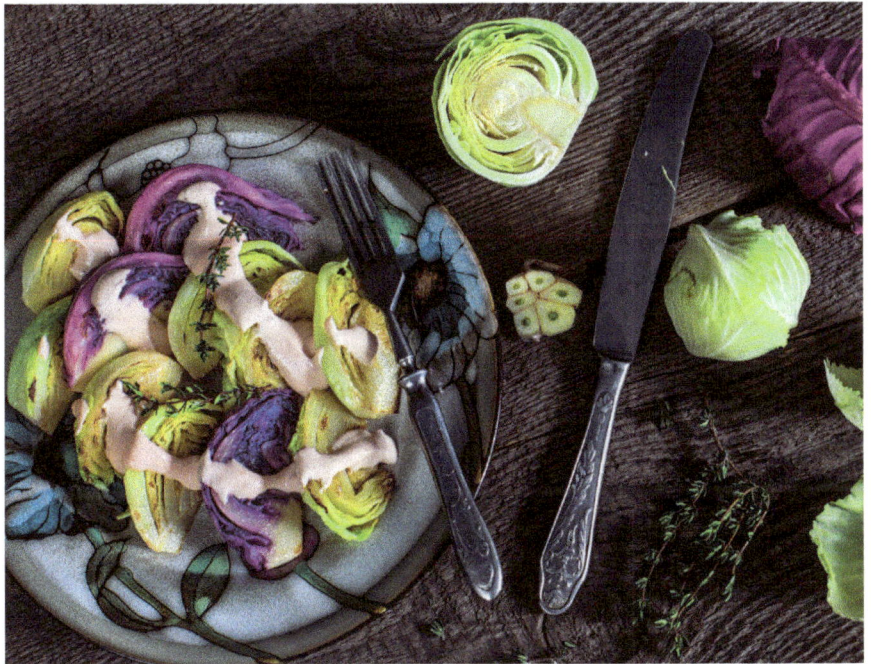

## Ingredients:

- 1 head cabbage, sliced into six 1-inch pieces
- 6 tablespoons olive oil
- salt and ground black pepper to taste

## Directions:

### Step 1

Preheat oven to 425 degrees F (220 degrees C).

### Step 2

Brush each cabbage piece on both sides with olive oil and season with salt and black pepper. Arrange in a single layer on a baking sheet.

### Step 3

Bake in the preheated oven until tender, 40 to 55 minutes.

Per Serving: 169 calories; protein 2.5g; carbohydrates 11.4g; fat 13.7g; sodium 61.5mg.

# 46 - Balsamic Grilled Zucchini

| Preparation | Cooking | Servings |
|:---:|:---:|:---:|
| 10 min | 10 min | 4 |

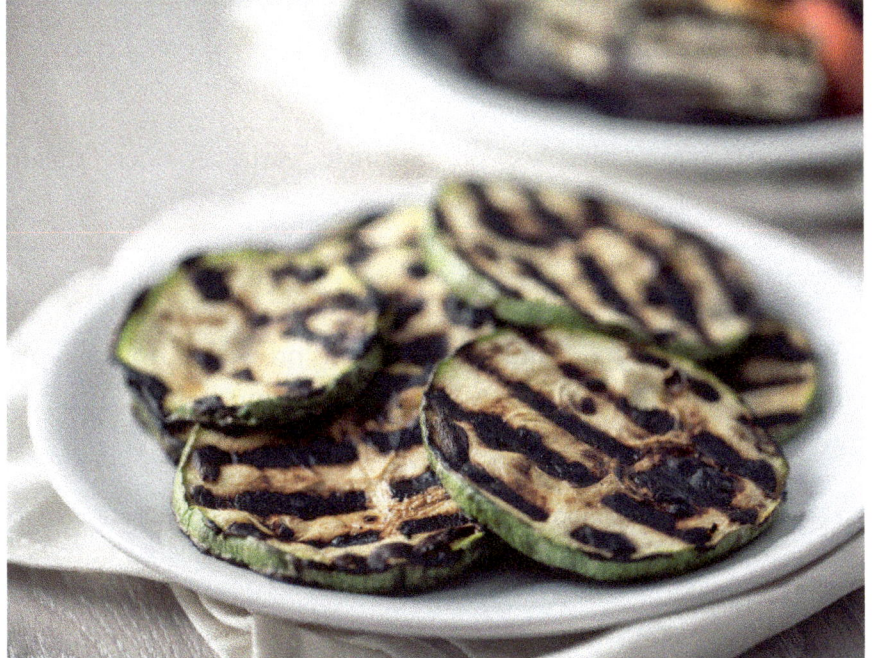

## Ingredients:

- 2 zucchinis, quartered lengthwise
- 2 teaspoons olive oil
- $\frac{1}{2}$ teaspoon garlic powder
- 1 teaspoon Italian seasoning

- 1 pinch salt

- 2 tablespoons balsamic vinegar

### Directions:

### Step 1

Preheat grill for medium-low heat and lightly oil the grate.

### Step 2

Brush zucchini with olive oil. Sprinkle garlic powder, Italian seasoning, and salt over zucchini.

### Step 3

Cook on preheated grill until beginning to brown, 3-4 minutes per side. Brush balsamic vinegar over the zucchini and continue cooking 1 minute more. Serve immediately.

**Per Serving: 38 calories; protein 0.8g; carbohydrates 3.6g; fat 2.5g; sodium 8mg.**

# 47 - Grilled Cauliflower

| Preparation | Cooking | Servings |
|:---:|:---:|:---:|
| 10 min | 20 min | 4 |

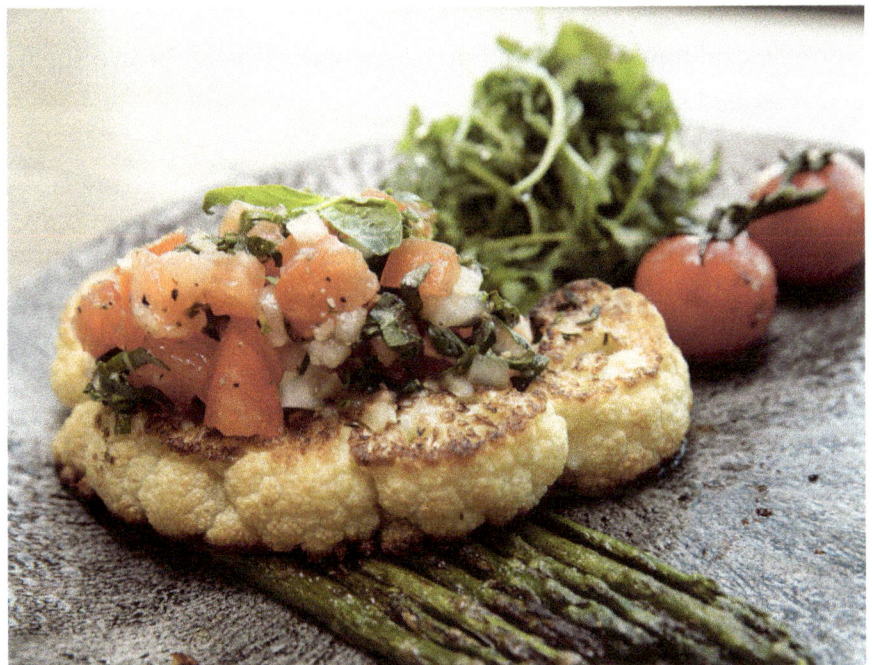

## Ingredients:

- 1 head cauliflower, cut into thick slices
- 1 tablespoon olive oil
- 1 tablespoon brown sugar
- 2 teaspoons seasoned salt

## Directions:

### Step 1

Preheat an outdoor grill for medium-high heat and lightly oil the grate.

### Step 2

Sprinkle cauliflower slices on both sides with olive oil, brown sugar, and seasoned salt.

### Step 3

Cook cauliflower on the grill until char marks appear, 2 to 3 minutes per side. Transfer to a grill-safe pan with a lid, cover, and continue cooking on grill until tender, about 20 minutes.

**Per Serving: 81 calories; protein 2.9g; carbohydrates 11.5g; fat 3.6g; sodium 502.9mg.**

# 48 – Grilled Yellow Squash

| Preparation | Cooking | Servings |
|:---:|:---:|:---:|
| 10 min | 20 min | 6 |

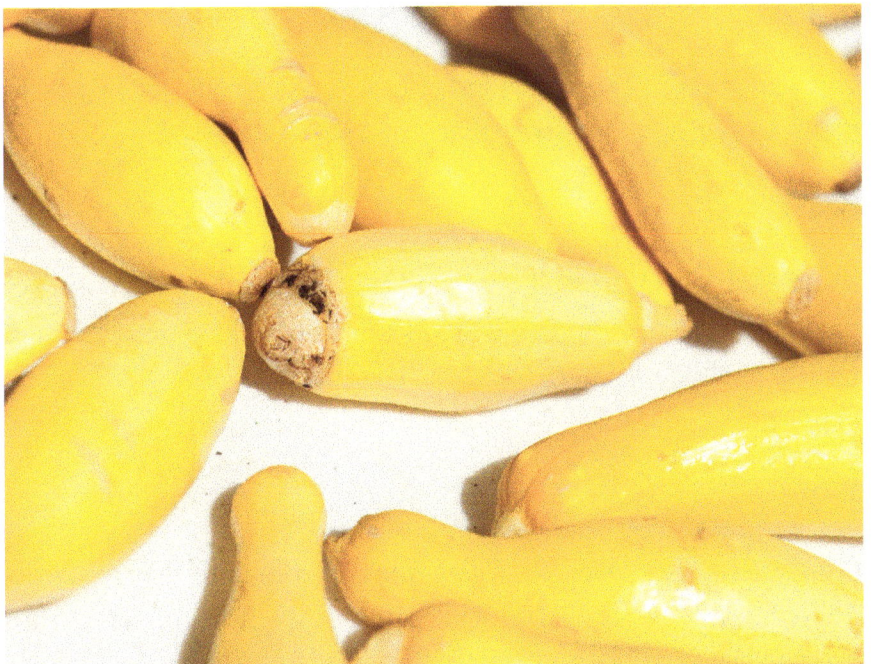

## Ingredients:

- 4 medium yellow squash
- $\frac{1}{2}$ cup extra virgin olive oil
- 2 cloves garlic, crushed
- salt and pepper to taste

## Directions:

### Step 1

Preheat the grill for medium heat.

### Step 2

Cut the squash horizontally into 1/4 inch to 1/2-inch-thick slices so that you have nice long strips that won't fall through the grill.

### Step 3

Heat olive oil in a small pan, and add garlic cloves. Cook over medium heat until the garlic starts to sizzle and become fragrant. Brush the slices of squash with the garlic oil, and season with salt and pepper.

### Step 4

Grill squash slices for 5 to 10 minutes per side, until they reach the desired tenderness. Brush with additional garlic oil, and turn occasionally to prevent sticking or burning.

Per Serving: 146 calories; protein 1g; carbohydrates 4.2g; fat 14.2g; sodium 2.1mg.

# 49 – Grilled Corn Salad

| Preparation | Cooking | Servings |
|:---:|:---:|:---:|
| 15 min | 10 min | 6 |

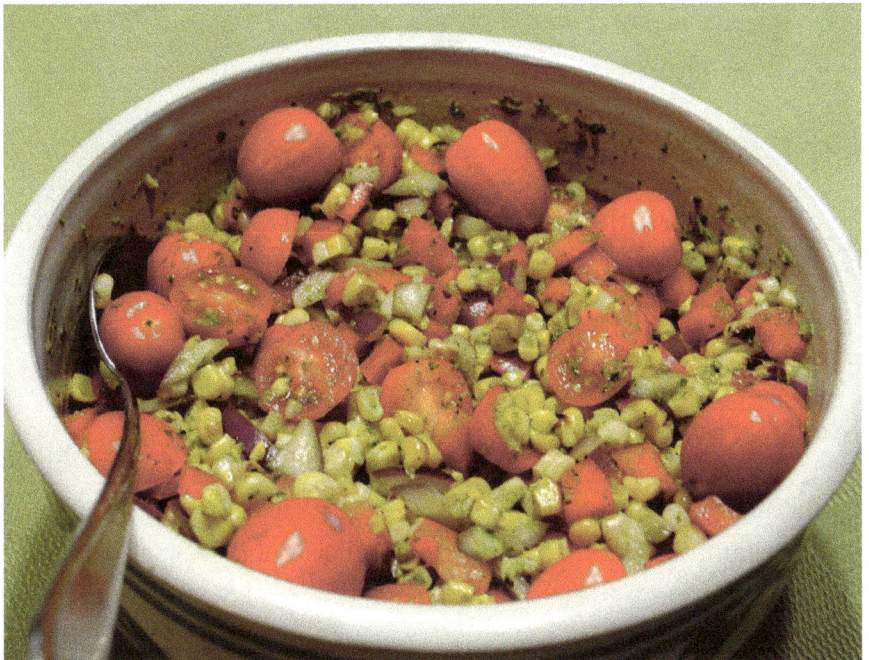

## Ingredients:

- 6 ears freshly shucked corn
- 1 green pepper, diced
- 2 Roma (plum) tomatoes, diced
- $\frac{1}{4}$ cup diced red onion

- $\frac{1}{2}$ bunch fresh cilantro, chopped, or more to taste

- 2 teaspoons olive oil, or to taste

- salt and ground black pepper to taste

### Directions:

### Step 1

Preheat an outdoor grill for medium heat; lightly oil the grate.

### Step 2

Cook the corn on the preheated grill, turning occasionally, until the corn is tender and specks of black appear, about 10 minutes; set aside until just cool enough to handle. Slice the kernels off of the cob and place into a bowl.

### Step 3

Combine the warm corn kernels with the green pepper, diced tomato, onion, cilantro, and olive oil. Season with salt and pepper; toss until evenly mixed. Set aside for at least 30 minutes to allow flavors to blend before serving.

Per Serving: 103 calories; protein 3.4g; carbohydrates 19.7g; fat 2.8g; sodium 43.4mg.

# 50 – Grilled Garlic Artichokes

| Preparation | Cooking | Servings |
|:---:|:---:|:---:|
| 15 min | 30 min | 4 |

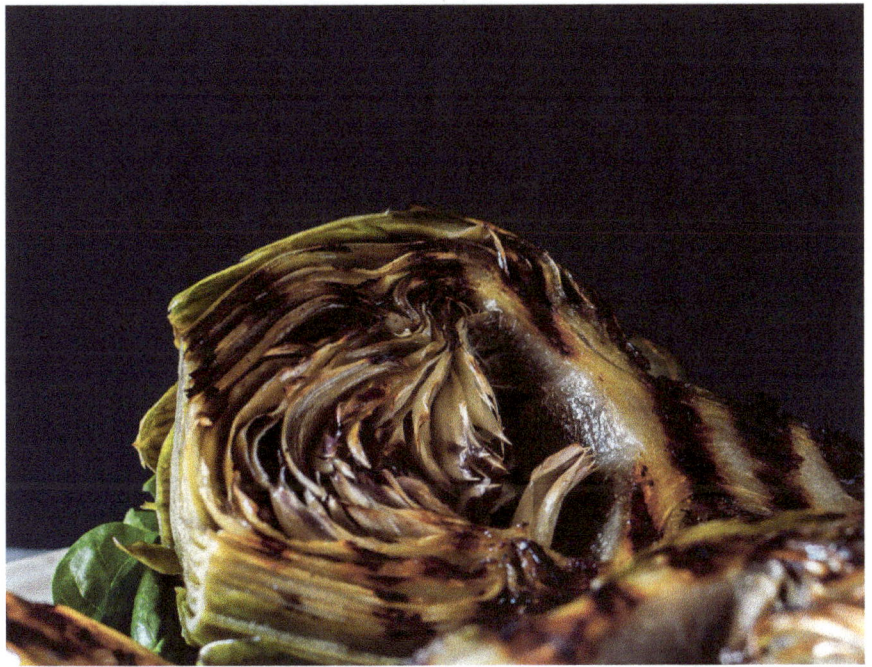

## Ingredients:

- 2 large artichokes
- 1 lemon, quartered
- $\frac{3}{4}$ cup olive oil
- 4 cloves garlic, chopped

- 1 teaspoon salt

- $\frac{1}{2}$ teaspoon ground black pepper

## Direction:

### Step 1

Fill a large bowl with cold water. Squeeze the juice from one lemon wedge into the water. Trim the tops from the artichokes, then cut in half lengthwise, and place halves into the bowl of lemon water to prevent them from turning brown.

### Step 2

Bring a large pot of water to a boil. Meanwhile, preheat an outdoor grill for medium-high heat.

### Step 3

Add artichokes to boiling water, and cook for about 15 minutes. Drain. Squeeze the remaining lemon wedges into a medium bowl. Stir in the olive oil and garlic, and season with salt and pepper.

### Step 4

Brush the artichokes with a coating of the garlic dip, and place them on the preheated grill. Grill the artichokes for 5 to 10 minutes, basting with dip and turning frequently, until the tips are a little charred. Serve immediately with the remaining dip.

Per Serving: 402 calories; protein 2.9g; carbohydrates 10g; fat 40.7g; sodium 659mg.

Lightning Source UK Ltd.
Milton Keynes UK
UKHW021119150421
382034UK00006B/62